OXFORD MEDICAL PUBLICATIONS

Effects of Smoking on the Fetus,
Neonate, and Child

This publication represents the proceedings of a symposium 'Effects of Smoking on the Fetus, Neonate and Child' held on 9–11 July 1990 at the Ciba Foundation, 41 Portland Place, London, W1N 4BN, and sponsored by the UK Department of Health, Hannibal House, London, SE1 6TE.

# Effects of Smoking on the Fetus, Neonate, and Child

Edited by

David Poswillo
*United Medical and Dental Schools*
*of Guy's and St Thomas' Hospitals*

and

Eva Alberman
*St Bartholomew's Medical College*

Oxford   New York   Tokyo
OXFORD UNIVERSITY PRESS
1992

Oxford University Press, Walton Street, Oxford OX2 6DP
Oxford   New York   Toronto
Delhi   Bombay   Calcutta   Madras   Karachi
Petaling Jaya   Singapore   Hong Kong   Tokyo
Nairobi   Dar es Salaam   Cape Town
Melbourne   Auckland
and associated companies in
Berlin   Ibadan

Oxford is a trade mark of Oxford University Press

Published in the United States
by Oxford University Press, New York

A catalogue record for this book is available from the British Library

Library of Congress Cataloging in Publication Data
Effects of smoking on the fetus, neonate, and child / edited by David
Poswillo and Eva Alberman.
p.    cm.—(Oxford medical publications)
Proceedings of a symposium held 9–11 July 1990 at the Ciba
Foundation, London, sponsored by the UK Dept. of Health.
Includes bibliographical references and index.
1. Pregnant women—Tobacco use—Health aspects—Congresses.
2. Fetus—Effect of chemicals on—Congresses.   3. Smoking—
Prevention—Congresses.   4. Passive smoking in infants—Congresses.
5. Passive smoking in children—Congresses.   I. Poswillo, David E.,
1927–  .   II. Alberman, Eva D. (Eva Dorothea)   III. Great Britain.
Dept. of Health.   IV. Series.
[DNLM: 1. Fetus—drug effects—congresses.   2. Maternal-Fetal
Exchange—congresses.   3. Pregnancy Complications—etiology—
congresses.   4. Smoking—adverse effects—congresses.   5. Smoking—
in pregnancy—congresses.   6. Tobacco Smoke Pollution—adverse
effects.    QV 137 E275 1990]
RG627.6.T6E33    1992.    618.3—dc20    92–13005
ISBN 0–19–262260–9

Typeset by Footnote Graphics, Warminster, Wiltshire
Printed and bound in Great Britain by
Bookcraft (Bath) Ltd, Midsomer Norton, Avon

# Foreword

This book has been produced as a result of the third international symposium organized by the Independent Scientific Committee on Smoking and Health: the first (*Nicotine, Smoking, and the Low Tar Programme*; Wald and Froggatt 1989) was published in 1989 and the second (*Smoking and Hormone-Related Disorders*; Wald and Baron 1990) in 1990. The Committee is grateful to David Poswillo, one of its members, and Eva Alberman for their skilful editing of this book, and the Department of Health for its help in funding the symposium and this publication.

The Committee was established in 1973 to provide unbiased advice to Health Ministers, and on occasions also the tobacco industry, on the scientific aspects of smoking and health. This advice depends *inter alia* on its comprehensiveness and for the past ten years we have sponsored a wide research programme using funds made available by the industry through the Tobacco Advisory Council and administered by the Committee's instrument, the Tobacco Products Research Trust. This programme has been directed mainly to the relationship between smoking-related diseases and the constitution of tobacco products in line with the terms of the 1980 'voluntary agreement' (between the industry and Government) through which the research funds were given (Independent Scientific Committee on Smoking and Health 1988). Generous as these terms are they do not cover all areas of our concern and we have chosen to augment our knowledge, on which our advice is based, by the international symposia referred to above. The knowledge thus gained has added greatly to the value of this advice.

We have plans for further symposia even though the EC Directives in the field of smoking and tobacco products make the future of national regulatory arrangements uncertain. Without these the Committee cannot formulate advice of the calibre that its brief would dictate, society would expect, and the public health require. 'Europe' in fact makes these desiderata all the more urgent and important, not less. It is a current challenge to the Committee to redefine its objectives within a European dimension and position itself to assume a role in improving the public health of the European Community as it has done in the United Kingdom.

Peter Froggatt
*Chairman, Independent Scientific Committee on*
*Smoking and Health and of the Tobacco Products*
*Research Trust*

# References

Independent Scientific Committee on Smoking and Health (1988). *Fourth Report.* HMSO, London.

Wald, N. and Baron, J. (ed.) (1990). *Smoking and Hormone-Related Disorders.* Oxford University Press, Oxford.

Wald, N. and Froggatt, P. (ed.) (1989). *Nicotine, Smoking, and the Low-Tar Programme.* Oxford University Press, Oxford.

# Contents

# Contributors

*Eva Alberman*
Wolfson Institute of Preventive Medicine, St Bartholomew's Medical College, London

*H Ross Anderson*
Department of Public Health Sciences, St George's Hospital Medical School, London

*Donna Day Baird*
Epidemiology Branch, National Institute of Environmental Health Sciences, North Carolina, USA

*J Martin Bland*
Department of Public Health Sciences, St George's Hospital Medical School, London

*Kulwinder S Bnait*
Department of Medical and Molecular Genetics, United Medical and Dental Schools of Guy's and St Thomas's Hospitals, London

*Graham J Burton*
Department of Anatomy, University of Cambridge, Cambridge

*Nigel J Cairns*
Department of Neuropathology, Institute of Psychiatry, London

*Oona Campbell*
Maternal and Child Epidemiology Unit, London School of Hygiene and Tropical Medicine, London

*Julie-Ann Evans*
Institute of Child Health, Royal Hospital for Sick Children, Bristol

*Frank A Fairweather*
Unilever, London

*R Louise Floyd*
Centers for Disease Control, Center for Chronic Disease Prevention and Health Promotion, Atlanta, USA

Pamela Gillies

Department of Public Health Medicine and Epidemiology, University Hospital and Medical School, Nottingham

Jean Golding

Institute of Child Health, Royal Hospital for Sick Children, Bristol

Eileen Gunter

Centers for Disease Control, Center for Chronic Disease Prevention and Health Promotion, Atlanta, USA

James E Haddow

Foundation for Blood Research, Maine, USA

Marion H Hall

Department of Obstetrics and Gynaecology, University of Aberdeen, Aberdeen

Valerie Harper

Department of Obstetrics and Gynaecology, University of Aberdeen, Aberdeen

Carol Hogue

Centers for Disease Control, Center for Chronic Disease Prevention and Health Promotion, Atlanta, USA

Julliette Kendrick

Centers for Disease Control, Center for Chronic Disease Prevention and Health Promotion, Atlanta, USA

George J Knight

Foundation for Blood Research, Maine, USA

George Knox

Department of Public Health and Epidemiology, Birmingham University Medical School, Birmingham

Christine MacArthur

Department of Public Health and Epidemiology, Birmingham University Medical School, Birmingham

James Marks

Centers for Disease Control, Center for Chronic Disease Prevention and Health Promotion, Atlanta, USA

Jon Nicholl

Medical Care Research Unit, Department of Public Health Medicine, University of Sheffield Medical School, Sheffield

*Alicia O'Cathain*
South Derbyshire Health Authority, Derby

*Glenn E Palomaki*
Foundation for Blood Research, Maine, USA

*Janet L Peacock*
Department of Public Health Sciences, St George's Hospital Medical School, London

*Jonathan Pollock*
Department of Child Health, University of Bristol, Bristol

*David Poswillo*
Department of Oral and Maxillofacial Surgery, United Medical and Dental Schools of Guy's and St Thomas's Hospitals, London

*David Rush*
USDA Human Nutrition Research Center on Aging at Tufts University, Boston, USA

*Mary J Seller*
Department of Medical and Molecular Genetics, United Medical and Dental Schools of Guy's and St Thomas's Hospitals, London

*Judy Stevens*
Centers for Disease Control, Center for Chronic Disease Prevention and Health Promotion, Atlanta, USA

*E Malcolm Symonds*
Department of Obstetrics and Gynaecology, University Hospital, Nottingham

*Robert Waller*
Department of Health, London

*Christine Zahniser*
Centers for Disease Control, Center for Chronic Disease Prevention and Health Promotion, Atlanta, USA

# 1. Introduction to toxicity

*Frank A Fairweather*

Toxicology, whether in relation to therapeutics, food, pesticides, the environment, occupational health, or indeed smoking, has come to mean that if a chemical compound produces a biological response within a living system, and that response is deemed hazardous, then the cause of this effect should be sought and where possible eliminated.   *Smoking can be seen in this aspect*

Clearly, for a chemical agent to produce such an effect in a biological system, there is a need for the toxic substance or its metabolites to reach an end organ, at a sufficiently high concentration and for an extended period of time, to produce the observed toxic response.

These principles, accepted now for many centuries, must be applied today when considering any potentially toxic material. It is the responsibility of all involved in the toxicological field to minimize the risk, to strive to ensure the acceptance of the doctrine that the better the decision, the better it is for the individual who will be exposed to the agent in question. Toxicology is now accepted as an integral part of the regulatory scene and it has become an intrinsic part of business. With respect to the latter it is refreshing to realize that test results can have a significant effect on marketing questions and toxicologists are now seeking to interpret adverse effects observed in animals and establish their relevance to humans.

There are certain points that, although well known, bear repetition. The mechanism of toxic response needs consideration in the context of smoking and its effects in pregnancy. The question of exposure to a toxic agent in relation to the mode of entry is highly relevant. The pharmacokinetics and metabolism must be considered in relation to the biochemical or indeed pathological lesion that may result. There may not always be a frank indication of such a prominent lesion but the cellular response to a noxious agent with its potential physiological consequences must be borne in mind and recognized.

The toxicity of any chemical must be considered in relation to the conditions of exposure. This includes consideration of such issues as the frequency of exposure, the dose that is actually delivered, the route by which the material enters the biological system and the all-important physical and chemical forms of the substance being administered.

Exposure may be acute or chronic. In the first instance the dose is usually given on one occasion and the absorption of the material is rapid. The effects of this will be seen in a short time. However, frequent bursts of acute exposure may lead to chronic effects. On the other hand, chronic exposure, where the compound is delivered with some frequency over a long period of time, will result in long-term ill-effects, these being determined by the dose of the material administered and the inherent toxicity of that compound. Also, in considering chronic toxicity, it is important to bear in mind the route of administration of the material because a spectrum of toxic effects may be seen when comparing, as an example, the inhalational route to the oral or dermal.

In seeking to recognize the factors that influence toxicity it is cogent to appreciate those that are within the toxic agent itself, and those that are widely related to exposure. However, consideration must also be given to those environmental factors that may play synergistic effects in producing in the 'end organ' a pathological effect or lead to physical consequences.

Having established some toxicological principles, the question of exposure of the fetus, neonate, and child to tobacco smoke is considered. Cigarette smoke is composed of some 3000 different compounds (Abel 1980) and the main components to be considered are carbon monoxide, nicotine, polycyclic aromatic hydrocarbons (PAHs), and others such as cyanide and cadmium.

Workers in this field agree that although these substances in some way affect the smoker, the pharmacological response seen in the smoker is primarily due to nicotine (Kelly *et al.* 1984). As smokers inhale the bolus of smoke that is formed in the mouth, a complex mixture of chemical compounds is taken in, which may simply be broken down into two fractions. The first consists of the PAHs—particulate matter that carries the nicotine into the lung suspended on its particles. The second fraction is known as the gaseous phase, and consists of carbon monoxide, oxides of nitrogen, hydrogen, cyanide, and several other constituents (Jaffe 1980; Taylor 1980).

These components of tobacco smoke have been associated with the diseases of smoking for some time, but over the last decade the substances have been highlighted as being those that produce various effects during pregnancy (Bottoms *et al.* 1982; Harrison *et al.* 1983; Luck *et al.* 1985).

At the conclusion of an excellent monograph, *Tobacco smoking*, the International Agency for Research on Cancer (IARC), concludes:

Tobacco smoke affects not only people who smoke but also people who are exposed to the combustion products of other people's tobacco. The effects produced are not necessarily the same, as the constituents of smoke vary according to its source. Three main sources exist: (i) mainstream smoke, (ii) sidestream smoke, and (iii) smoke exhaled to the general atmosphere by smokers. Smokers are exposed to all three to a greater extent than are non-smokers. It follows that it is unlikely that any effects will be produced in passive smokers that are not produced to a greater extent in smokers and that types of effects that are not seen in smokers will not be seen in passive smokers. Examination of smoke from the different sources shows that all three types contain chemicals that are both carcinogenic and mutagenic. The amounts absorbed by passive smokers are, however, small and effects are unlikely to be detectable unless exposure is substantial and very large numbers of people are observed. The observations on non-smokers that have been made so far are compatible with either an increased risk from 'passive' smoking or an absence of risk. Knowledge of the nature of sidestream and mainstream smoke, of the materials absorbed during 'passive' smoking, and of the quantitative relationships between dose and effect that are commonly observed from exposure to carcinogens, however, leads to the conclusion that passive smoking gives rise to some risk of cancer. *→7 figures of women.*

**Evaluations**

There is sufficient evidence that inhalation of tobacco smoke as well as topical applications of tobacco smoke condensate cause cancer in experimental animals.

There is sufficient evidence that tobacco smoke is carcinogenic to humans.

The occurrence of malignant tumours of the respiratory tract and of the upper digestive tract is causally related to the smoking of different forms of tobacco (cigarettes, cigars, pipes, bidis). The occurrence of malignant tumours of the bladder, renal pelvis and pancreas is causally related to the smoking of cigarettes (IARC 1986).

It is a matter of deep regret that there appears to be no comment on transplacental passage and risk. From the toxicological point of view it is difficult to identify one material that could be producing cellular damage eventually leading to disease. As has been stressed, tobacco smoke is a combined cocktail of chemicals, some probably causing more damage than others, and includes such chemicals as acrolein, cadmium, formaldehyde, nitrosamines, oxide of nitrogen, and many others.

Against this background can be considered the physical consequences of this effect of smoking, which in this case may include such issues as low birth weight, congenital malformations, learning disorders and decreased intelligence, increase in still birth and neonatal deaths, and an increase in spontaneous abortion and placenta praevia.

In summary, it is clear that cigarette smoking and its effects on the fetus, neonate, and child is a complex subject. Toxicology is a multidisciplinary subject and it is for this reason that one can only plead that if knowledge of this all-important field is to be furthered, all disciplines need to move forward in harmony, because many factors must be assessed to clarify this issue. The following chapters will address these issues.

# References

Abel, E. L. (1980). Smoking during pregnancy—a review of effects on growth and development of offspring. *Human Biology,* **52,** 593–625.

Bottoms, S. F., Kuhnert, B. R., Kuhnert, P. M., and Reese, A. L. (1982). Maternal passive smoking and fetal thiocyanate levels. *American Journal of Obstetrics and Gynecology,* **144,** 787–91.

Harrison, G., Branson, R. S., and Vaucher, Y. E. (1983). Association of maternal smoking with body composition of the newborn. *American Journal of Clinical Nutrition,* **38,** 757–62.

International Agency for Research on Cancer (IARC) (1986). Monograph on the Evaluation of the Carcinogenic Risk of Chemicals to Humans. *Tobacco Smoking,* vol. 38, p. 314. IARC, Lyon.

Jaffe, J. H. (1980). *Drug addiction and drug abuse*. In *The pharmacological basis of therapeutics*, (ed. A. G. Gilman, L. Goodman, and A. Gilman), pp. 535–60. Macmillan Publishing Company Incorporated, New York.

Kelly, J., Mathews, K. A., and O'Conor, M. (1984). Smoking in pregnancy: effects on mother and fetus. *British Journal of Obstetrics and Gynaecology*, **91,** 111–17.

Luck, W., Nau, H., Hansen, R., and Steldinger, R. (1985). Extent of nicotine and cotinine transfer to the fetus, placenta and amniotic fluid of smoking mothers. *Developmental Pharmacology and Therapeutics*, **8,** 384–95.

Taylor, P. (1980). *Ganglionic stimulating and blocking agents*. In *The pharmacological basis of therapeutics*, (ed. A. G. Gilman, L. S. Goodman, and A. Gilman), pp. 211–20. Macmillan Publishing Company Incorporated, New York.

# 2. Evidence for reduced fecundity in female smokers

*Donna Day Baird*

## Introduction

Cigarette smoking has been linked with several adverse reproductive outcomes (Rosenberg 1987). The most consistently reported effect is reduction in birth weight (reviewed by Hogue and Sappenfield 1987). The question of whether smoking adversely affects a woman's ability to become pregnant has received less attention. Data on smoking and fertility are available from several epidemiological studies, but only one of these was designed specifically to address this question. In a 1986 review article on the subject, Stillman *et al.* (1986) claimed that: 'this literature clearly demonstrates a reduction in fecundity of women who smoke.' Yet, in the accompanying editorial, Wentz (1986) stated: 'There are few good hard data that show that smoking impairs fertility. Published data are weighted in the direction of showing no deleterious effect on fertility in the woman.' Clearly a controversy existed. Additional reports published after 1986 do not resolve this controversy.

The purpose of this chapter is to evaluate the evidence for a causal relationship between cigarette smoking and subfecundity in women. Fecundity is defined here as the biological ability to become pregnant, and to maintain the pregnancy long enough for it to be clinically detected. Thus, a woman must be able to ovulate viable ova and provide the supportive environment for fertilization, implantation, and early development. The chapter includes a critical review of the existing epidemiological data and a consideration of the biological plausibility for an adverse effect of smoking. Specific issues are identified that need further research to clarify the currently available data. Finally, considering the current data, what public health recommendations are warranted?

## Epidemiological studies

Data on smoking and fecundity have been reported from 15 epidemiological studies. They include cross-sectional, prospective, and case-control studies, and they vary in the selectivity of their participants, and in their measures of fecundity and smoking (Table 2.1).

The findings regarding smoking in several of the studies of fecundity must

**Table 2.1** Literature review of studies including data on female smoking and fecundity, ordered by year of publication

| First author and date | Study design | Participants | Measurement of fecundity | Measurement of smoking | Estimated RR of infertility for smokers[1] | Control for potential confounders |
|---|---|---|---|---|---|---|
| Tokuhata (1968) | Cross-sectional analysis of participants in case-control study | 2016 married women who died 1950–1967 569 breast cancers 921 controls matched on race, year of death, age of death | Ever/never pregnant | Ever smoke during lifetime | 1.5 | Cause of death, age, race, occupation, education, year of death, number of marriages; husband's smoking, education, occupation |
| Mai et al. (1972) | Case-control | 50 infertile cases (seeking treatment at infertility clinic) 50 fertile controls (selected from hospital clinics or acquaintance of cases) Attempt to frequency match on age, SES, religion, country of origin, years married, age difference between spouses | Seeking treatment for infertility | Smoking status at time of study | More heavy smokers among infertile | Matching variables |

| Reference | Design | Population | Outcome | Exposure measure | Result | Confounders adjusted |
|---|---|---|---|---|---|---|
| Freidman (1977) | Prospective (insemination treatments) | 227 women receiving artificial donor insemination | Pregnant or not during AID treatment | Not reported; probably smoking status at treatment | No significant influence | None |
| Linn et al. (1982) | Cross-sectional | 3214 post partum married women who stopped using contraception in order to conceive, excluding those with surgery or drug treatment for infertility, diabetes, or multiple births; selected from 7676 interviewed women | >3 months to conceive versus ≤ 3 months | Smoking status during pregnancy | 1.0 (0.9, 1.2) | Age, race, income, education, body mass, type contraception, religion, prenatal DES, age of menarche, pregnancy history, marijuana use, history of pelvic inflammatory disease |
| Olsen et al. (1983) | Case-control | 437 infertility cases (excluding male-factor infertility); 2969 controls who conceived within a year (excluded women with diabetes, arthritis, goitre, cancer and thyroid disorders) | Seeking treatment for infertility | Smoking status during year of most recent pregnancy | 2.3 (1.8–2.9) | Age, education, oral contraceptive use anytime before attempted pregnancy, pregnancy history, history of infertility, alcohol |

**Table 2.1** (*Continued*)

| First author and date | Study design | Participants | Measurement of fecundity | Measurement of smoking | Estimated RR of infertility for smokers[1] | Control for potential confounders |
|---|---|---|---|---|---|---|
| Olsen *et al.* (1983) | Case-control | 423 case pregnancies that required a year or more to conceive; 3200 control pregnancies conceived within a year (excluded women with diabetes, arthritis, goitre, cancer and thyroid disorders) | Requiring more than 12 months to conceive | Smoking status during year of most recent pregnancy | 1.6 (1.2–2.0) | Age, education, oral contraceptive use anytime before attempted pregnancy, pregnancy history, history of infertility, alcohol |
| Harlap and Baras (1984) | Cross-sectional | 5880 women, 1-day postpartum, who desired pregnancy and stopped contraception in order to conceive; selected from 16 583 postpartum women | Time to pregnancy in months | Not reported; probably smoking status postpartum | No effect on fertility | Type of contraception |
| Stubblefield *et al.* (1984) | Prospective (follow-up questionnaire every 3 months) | 1112 women who had unprotected intercourse at least once during a 3-month follow-up period | Pregnancy rate (number of pregnancies per month of follow-up) | Smoking status at enrolment | No apparent association | Year enroled, age, race, marital status, religion, body mass, age of menarche, type of contraception, |

| Baird and Wilcox (1985) | Cross-sectional | 678 married pregnant women with planned pregnancies who conceived within two years | Time to pregnancy (number of menstrual cycles) | Smoking status at beginning of time to pregnancy | 2.1 | $P < 0.01$ | Age, income, education, employment status, frequency, of intercourse, oral contraceptive use, body mass, age of menarche, pregnancy history, alcohol, marijuana, history of pelvic inflammatory disease, method of recruitment, gestational age at interview | alcohol, coffee, aspirin, prescription drugs, gravidity, history of urinary tract infection, pelvic inflammatory disease |

**Table 2.1** (*Continued*)

| First author and date | Study design | Participants | Measurement of fecundity | Measurement of smoking | Estimated RR of infertility for smokers[1] | Control for potential confounders |
|---|---|---|---|---|---|---|
| Howe et al. (1985) | Prospective (follow-up each clinic visit or annually) | 4104 women stopping birth control in order to conceive; selected from 17 032 white, married women | Time to pregnancy (months to delivery adjusted for birth outcome) | Smoking status at enrolment | 1.2 *P* for trend < 0.001 | Age, social class, contraception, body mass, pregnancy history, reported gynaecological disorders, age at marriage |
| Daling et al. (1987) | Case-control | 170 primary tubal infertility patients; 170 controls who delivered a baby during year after case started trying to conceive matched on age, race, census tract | Seeking treatment for infertility | Smoking status at beginning of time to pregnancy | 2.7 (1.4–5.3) | Income, education, oral contraceptive use, IUD use, religion, number of sexual partners, first intercourse, douching habits, husband smoking |
| Hartz et al. (1987) | Cross-sectional | 35 973 white married women >30 years old (excluding ex-smokers); selected from 50 145 women age 20–59 who | Ever/never pregnant | Number of cigarettes/day at time of study | 1.3 | Age, obesity, husband's education |

| Study | Design | Sample | Outcome | Exposure | Results | Confounders considered |
|---|---|---|---|---|---|---|
| Phipps *et al.* (1987). | Case-control | 901 primary infertility cases; 1802 controls who delivered live-born babies, matched on age, race, payment status (excluded control women with history of infertility treatment) responded to a questionnaire mailed to 125 000 TOPS (Take Off Pounds Sensibly) members | Seeking treatment for infertility | Smoking status before started trying to conceive | Tubal (*n* = 283) 1.6 (1.1–2.1) Cervical (*n* =184) 1.5 (1.0–2.1) Ovulatory (*n* = 566) 1.2 (0.9–1.5) Endometriosis (*n* = 286) 1.0 (0.7–1.4) | Education, religion, any prior use of oral contraceptive, medical centre, time between menarche and attempt to conceive, IUD use, history of barrier methods of contraception, douching, menstrual irregularity before IUD use |
| deMouzon *et al.* (1988) | Prospective (temperature charts each menstrual cycle of trying) | 1887 volunteer couples without known fertility problems, currently trying to conceive | Time to pregnancy (number of menstrual cycles) | Smoking status at entry to study | 1.4 (not significant) | Age, income, frequency of intercourse, use of oral contraceptives, body mass, exercise, age of menarche, gravidity, history |

**Table 2.1** (*Continued*)

| First author and date | Study design | Participants | Measurement of fecundity | Measurement of smoking | Estimated RR of infertility for smokers[1] | Control for potential confounders |
|---|---|---|---|---|---|---|
| | | | | | | of spontaneous abortions, history of infertility, male smoking, started trying to conceive before entering study |
| Rowland (1989) | Cross-sectional | 436 registered dental assistants married, working full-time, pregnant during prior 4 years, pregnancy not due to birth control failure; selected from respondents to mail screener questionnaire (69% response rate to screener) | Time to pregnancy (number of menstrual cycles) | Smoking status at beginning to time to pregnancy | 1.9 $P = 0.06$ | Age, race, income, occupational exposures, frequency of intercourse, use of oral contraceptives, body mass, exercise, pelvic inflammatory disease, sexually transmitted diseases, number of sexual partners, pregnancy history, spouse smoking |

| Hatch (1990) | Cross-sectional | 1909 married women recruited from prenatal clinics, ≥ 18 years old, and stopped birth control at an identifiable time before pregnancy (selected from target population of 6219) | Time to pregnancy (number of months) | Average number of cigarettes/ day for 12 months before pregnancy | < 1.0 (not significant) | Age, race, education, oral contraceptive use, pregnancy history, age at menarche, medical history, DES, IUD use, caffeine, alcohol, and marijuana use |

[1] Infertility is defined somewhat differently in each of these studies so the relative risk estimates are not strictly comparable. In Tokuhata (1968), the value is the relative risk of having never been pregnant. In Linn *et al.* (1982) the value is the relative risk of taking more than 3 months to conceive. In Olsen *et al.* (1983), Daling *et al.* (1987), and Phipps *et al.* (1987) the value is the odds ratio for cases compared to controls. For Baird and Wilcox (1985), deMouzon *et al.* (1988), and Rowland (1989) the relative risk of taking more than 12 menstrual cycles to conceive, calculated from the per cycle fecundability ratio. The values for Howe *et al.* (1985) and Hatch (1990) are the relative risk of taking more than 12 months to conceive, crudely estimated from the fecundability ratios provided in the paper.

be discounted because of serious limitations in data collection, analysis, or reporting. The earliest case-control study (Mai *et al.* 1972) was small (50 infertile cases and 50 controls) and smoking was not a focus of the study. The study reported more heavy smokers in the infertile group, but provided no additional information. In addition, they recruited hospital or friend controls, which would tend to bias results towards the null.

Findings from two cross-sectional analyses (Tokuhata 1968; Hartz *et al.* 1987) are also questionable because of the crudeness of the smoking and fecundity data (neither study was designed specifically to look at this relationship). Hartz *et al.* (1987) collected data on number of cigarettes smoked per day at the time of study rather than at the time when the woman was trying to become pregnant. Tokuhata (1968) categorized women as smokers if they had ever smoked regularly at any time in their lives. In both studies fecundity was measured by ever/never pregnant, without information on desire for pregnancy. In addition, Tokuhata's data were collected from relatives or friends, rather than from the identified subject.

Findings regarding smoking and fecundity in three of the four prospective studies also present serious problems of interpretation. The earliest prospective study (Friedman 1977) described the experience of a group of 227 women treated with artificial insemination by donor. The author reported 'no significant influence' of smoking on pregnancy rates in this group. No other information is given. Aside from potential misclassification of smoking status (smokers who do not become pregnant in the first few menstrual cycles may stop smoking) and potential selection bias, the major problem is with the outcome variable (pregnant or not). Women who continued with therapy would be more likely eventually to become pregnant. Yet, there was no indication that this was taken into account in the analysis. If smokers were more likely than non-smokers to stop therapy after one or two unsuccessful insemination cycles, an adverse effect of smoking could be masked.

A second prospective study is also difficult to interpret. It was designed to evaluate the effects of induced abortion on future fecundity (Stubblefield *et al.* 1984). The authors included smoking habits in a multivariate analysis of 1112 women who were potentially at risk of becoming pregnant. 'No association' of smoking with the monthly pregnancy rate was found. However, analyses included women who stopped birth control completely in order to become pregnant, as well as women who were using birth control regularly except for one event. A smoking effect could be obscured if smokers were more likely than non-smokers to use birth control somewhat sporadically.

Conclusions from another prospective study must also be questioned (DeMouzon *et al.* 1988). The researchers enrolled women who were trying to conceive and followed their cycles to conception with daily basal body temperature measurements. Crude analysis showed significantly reduced pregnancy rates among smokers. Multivariate analysis showed a non-significant 14 per cent reduction in pregnancy rates associated with smoking. However, smokers were more likely to have begun trying to conceive before entering the study, and this was inappropriately controlled in the multivariate analysis by including a 'yes'/'no' variable for prior trying in the statistical model. Thus, some of the reduction in fecundity associated with smoking was assigned to another variable in the model.

The remaining nine studies have better analyses of smoking and fecundity. Six of these showed adverse effects on fecundity associated with smoking. These six include one prospective study (Howe *et al.* 1985), three case-control studies (Olsen *et al.* 1983; Daling *et al.* 1987; Phipps *et al.* 1987) and two cross-sectional studies (Baird and Wilcox 1985; Rowland 1989).

The three studies that found no effect of smoking on fecundity (Linn *et al.* 1982; Harlap and Baras 1984; Hatch 1990) are all large studies. Though none of these studies was designed to study smoking, there is no obvious methodological problem in any of them that would prevent an effect of smoking from appearing in the data if one were truly there. The biggest problem with these studies is possible bias from reporting errors. Each is a study of currently or very recently pregnant women. Fecundity was measured imprecisely as evidenced by substantial digit preference in data on time to pregnancy. Two of the three studies (Linn *et al.* 1982; Harlap and Baras 1984) collected data on smoking during pregnancy rather than during the time of trying to become pregnant. Resulting random misclassification of both smoking status and fecundity would probably bias results toward the null (Baird *et al.* 1991), but an adverse effect, if one exists, should still be apparent, given the large sample sizes in these studies.

A possible bias that could have masked a real effect of smoking in these three studies could have resulted from non-random reporting errors in time-to-pregnancy data. All three of these studies limited analysis to women who had stopped using birth control in order to become pregnant (a minority of each population being studied). Oral contraceptive use was a commonly reported method of birth control in all these studies. Because some doctors recommend that couples wait 3 to 6 months after stopping oral contraceptive use before trying to conceive, many women abstain, or use rhythm or a barrier method of contraception for a few months after oral contraceptive use. In interviewing women regarding their time to pregnancy, we found that many women will report 'pill' as their last method of birth control, even when they used another method to prevent pregnancy for an additional few months. This would tend to enhance the apparent adverse effect of pill use. If smokers are less likely than non-smokers to prevent pregnancy for a few months after stopping the pill, smoking will appear to be 'protective' of the artifactual reduction in fecundity associated with the pill-associated reporting errors. This could obscure a true adverse effect of smoking.

The studies that show a relationship between smoking and reduced fecundity (Olsen *et al.* 1983; Baird and Wilcox 1985; Howe *et al.* 1985; Daling *et al.* 1987; Phipps *et al.* 1987; Rowland 1989) can also be criticized on methodological grounds. Misclassification in smoking status and fecundity may have been a problem (see Table 2.1 for definitions of these variables in each study), but the resultant bias would be expected to mask an effect, rather than create one.

Potential confounding variables were not consistently controlled in these analyses, except for age and a measure of socio-economic level. Frequency of intercourse was analysed only by Baird and Wilcox (1985) and Rowland (1989). However, smokers and non-smokers were very similar in their frequency of intercourse, suggesting that this may not be a problem in the studies that did not collect these data. Though oral contraceptive use was not controlled in Olsen's or Phipp's analyses, it may not have biased results. These were case-control studies where pill use will be less important because its predominant effects on fecundity are short-term (Linn *et al.* 1982; Harlap and Baras 1984). Smoking habits of the male partner might also influence a couple's ability to conceive, but none of the three studies that examined this potential confounder found any association with reduced fecundity (Baird and Wilcox 1985; Daling *et al.* 1987; Rowland 1989). Three potential confounders have not been adequately controlled in any of the reviewed studies (caffeine intake, recreational drug use, and pelvic inflammatory disease). These will be discussed in the section on further research (p. 19).

The potential for selection bias in studies showing an association between smoking and fecundity is also problematic. Baird and Wilcox (1985) and Howe *et al.* (1985) analysed time to pregnancy only for planned pregnancies. As Baird and Wilcox point out, this might artifactually create a smoking effect if smokers are more likely to have accidental pregnancies. If, as one would expect, accidental pregnancies are more likely to occur in the most fecund women, highly fecund smokers will be selected out of the study to a greater extent than highly fecund non-smokers. The smokers remaining in the study will represent the less fecund subset of the target population of smokers. However, Baird and Wilcox (1985) estimated that this potential bias could only have explained a small portion of the smoking effect observed in their study. Two other data sources also suggest that this 'planning bias' cannot explain the findings. First, the potential bias should be weaker in Rowland's study (1989), because he studied all pregnancies except those due to actual birth control failure, yet the effect of smoking in his study is similar to that observed by Baird *et al.* Secondly, recent data suggest that smokers may not be more likely to have accidental pregnancies (Weller *et al.* 1987).

Case-control studies of women seeking infertility treatment are also subject to selection bias because a minority of couples who have trouble conceiving seek treatment. (Hirsch and Mosher (1987) estimate that only one-third of US couples seek treatment.) However, this potential selection bias does not appear to explain the observed smoking effect. First, if the effect was due only to selection (smokers being more likely to seek treatment than non-smokers), one would expect smoking to be associated with all types of infertility. However, in all these case-control studies smoking was most strongly associated with tubal infertility. Secondly, Olsen *et al.* (1983) included a second case group in their case-control study, women who tried for more than a year to conceive but did not seek infertility services. These cases were also significantly more likely to smoke than controls.

The most convincing epidemiological evidence for an adverse effect of smoking on fecundity is dose–response data. Dose–response information was provided in five of the six studies that reported a smoking effect (Baird and Wilcox 1985; Howe *et al.* 1985; Daling *et al.* 1987; Phipps *et al.* 1987; Rowland 1989). Data from all five are consistent with a dose response (Table 2.2). Such a pattern is unlikely to arise by chance in five separate studies. Systematic bias is also an unlikely cause of these patterns because the study designs of the five studies differ: one is prospective (Howe *et al.* 1985), two are cross-sectional (Baird *et al.* 1985; Rowland 1989), and two are case-control studies (Daling *et al.* 1987; Phipps *et al.* 1987).

**Table 2.2** Dose–response relationships reported for cigarette smoking and fecundity

| Author and date | Dose–response data with relative risks[1] | | Definition of infertility |
|---|---|---|---|
| Baird and Wilcox (1985) | Non-smokers | 1.0 | > 12 cycles to conceive |
| | 1–20 cigs/day | 1.9 | |
| | > 20 cigs/day | 2.9 | |
| Howe *et al.* (1985) | Never smokers | 1.0 | > 12 months to conceive |
| | 1–5 cigs/day | 1.0 | |
| | 6–10 cigs/day | 1.1 | |
| | 11–15 cigs/day | 1.2 | |
| | 16–20 cigs/day | 1.7 | |
| | > 20 cigs/day | 1.7 | |
| Daling *et al.* (1987) | Never smokers | 1.0 | Tubal infertility |
| | 1–10 cigs/day | 2.0 | |
| | > 10 cigs/day | 3.2 | |
| Phipps *et al.* (1987) | Never smokers | 1.0 | Tubal infertility |
| | < 5 pack years | 1.4 | |
| | ≥ 5 pack years | 1.6 | |
| Rowland (1989) | Non-smokers | 1.0 | > 12 cycles to conceive |
| | 10 cigs/day[2] | 1.9 | |
| | 20 cigs/day[2] | 2.8 | |

[1] Relative risks for infertility were calculated from fecundity ratios reported by Baird and Wilcox; Howe *et al.*, 1985; Rowland, 1989.

[2] The smoking variable in the multivariate model was number of cigarettes per day because it appeared to fit the data better than a dichotomized variable for smoking status. Thus, there is evidence for a dose relationship, but the relative risk estimates are forced by the model.

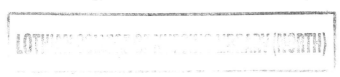

## Biological mechanisms

In laboratory animals, smoking can adversely influence several reproductive processes required for achieving clinically detectable pregnancy, including ovulation, tubal transport, pre-implantation development, and implantation (reviewed by Mattison 1982).

The extent to which these mechanisms operate in women is not known. Effects on pre-implantation development and implantation have not been studied. The few data that address the issue of ovarian function in smokers are mixed. The data supporting an effect are indirect. Menstrual cyclicity was reported to differ between smokers and non-smokers (Sloss and Frerichs 1983) and several epidemiological studies found earlier menopause in smokers (reviewed by Baron 1984). Also, oestrogen metabolism can be influenced by smoking, with smokers metabolizing more of their oestradiol to catechol forms (Michnovicz *et al.* 1986), which are quickly cleared and are inactive at most target sites. On the other hand, the only data comparing anovulation rates in smokers and non-smokers showed no difference between the two groups (MacMahon *et al.* 1982). In addition, both case-control studies of infertility patients in the US found no effects of smoking on ovulatory infertility (Daling *et al.* 1987; Phipps *et al.* 1987). However, as Phipps *et al.* note, this category of infertility included diverse pathologies such as luteal phase defect and polycystic ovary disease, so smoking may have been related to a portion of these pathologies without showing an overall effect.

Effects of smoking on tubal transport in women are suggested both by experimental and epidemiologic studies. The experimental work (reviewed by Phipps *et al.* 1987) indicates that smoking directly impairs tubal function and reduces immune response so that increased susceptibility to tubal damage by infectious agents could result. These findings are consistent with an association between smoking and tubal infertility, as found in three case-control studies of infertility (Olsen *et al.* 1983; Daling *et al.* 1987; Phipps *et al.* 1987).

However, if smoking impairs fecundity by increasing a woman's susceptibility to tubal damage from infectious agents, one would expect ex-smokers to show reduced fecundity as well as current smokers. None of the four studies that reported on fecundity of ex-smokers found adverse effects in ex-smokers (Baird and Wilcox 1985; Howe *et al.* 1985; Daling *et al.* 1987; Phipps *et al.* 1987). This argues against a strong role for an immunologically-mediated mechanism.

## Issues for further study

Despite the reported dose–response relationships and biological plausibility, a causal relationship between smoking and fecundity must still be considered tentative. The epidemiological studies do not consistently show adverse effects, and the estimated associations are relatively weak (RR (relative risk) = 1.2–2.8). A major concern is that a weak effect could result from un-measured confounding factors. Potential confounders in need of more careful assessment include consumption of caffeinated beverages, recreational drug use, and history of sexually transmitted diseases and pelvic inflammatory disease.

Wilcox *et al.* (1988) recently reported a strong dose–response relationship between caffeine consumption and fecundity. Hatch reports a similar finding (1990). An association was also found in preliminary analysis of another data set (Christianson *et al.* 1989). However, Joesoef *et al.* (1990) found no associa-tion in their analysis of a large data set, and there is evidence for an effect only at high levels in two other large data sets (Williams *et al.* 1990; J. Olsen, personal communication). Because smoking and caffeine consumption are correlated (Schreiber *et al.* 1988), it is at least theoretically possible that the reported associations between smoking and subfecundity are really due to caffeine consumption.

Experimental data suggest that marijuana and cocaine use might impair fecundity, but epidemiological data are difficult to collect. The one published study that reports an association (Mueller *et al.* 1990) has substantial meth-odological problems (Weinberg 1990). Because the prevalence of drug use and its association with smoking is not well known, it is difficult to evaluate the potential for confounding by these exposures.

Another risk factor for subfecundity that is difficult to measure adequately is history of sexually transmitted diseases. Their association with tubal infer-tility raises special concern, in that the smoking–subfecundity association is reported to be strongest for tubal disease. To further complicate the issue, sexually transmitted disease could be either a confounder or a factor in the causal pathway (if smoking affects immune response such that smokers are more susceptible to tubal damage by infectious agents). Several studies con-trolled for self-reported history of sexually transmitted disease or pelvic inflammatory disease and still found effects of smoking (Baird and Wilcox 1985; Howe *et al.* 1985; Daling *et al.* 1987; Rowland 1989), but non-symptomatic disease is still an uncontrolled factor in these studies.

## Public health significance

A causal relationship between smoking and reduced fecundity is supported by the dose–reponse relationships found in epidemiological studies and by the biological plausibility demonstrated in laboratory studies. Though questions remain and the evidence is tentative, the data strongly support the need to inform the public of this additional potential reproductive risk associated with smoking. The available epidemiological data suggest that adverse effects are reversible, so if women were to stop smoking they could probably expect their fecundity to return to normal levels.

Clinical infertility affects 10–20 per cent of couples (Rachootin and Olsen 1982; Hull *et al*. 1985; Rantala and Koskimies 1986; Mosher 1988). This array of conditions is not well understood medically, and aetiological factors have not been properly studied. Treatment is invasive and expensive. If smoking does increase the risk of infertility by two-fold, cessation could reduce its prevalence by as much as 10 per cent, resulting in substantial savings in personal and public resources.

Public education regarding the potential adverse effects of smoking on fecundity should be designed to counter possible misinterpretations. Though smoking probably reduces a woman's chances of conceiving in any given menstrual cycle, it is *not* a method of birth control. Even if smoking reduces a woman's per cycle probability of pregnancy by 30 per cent, as found by Baird and Wilcox (1985), about 75 per cent of sexually active smokers who did not use any method of contraception would still be expected to become pregnant within a year.

Finally, information about the potential adverse effects of smoking on fecundity could motivate some women to stop smoking. All women who smoke should be encouraged to stop, but those concerned about their fecundity may be a particularly receptive group. Health professionals who counsel these women should encourage them to stop smoking. Anti-smoking programmes directed at them might be particularly successful.

# References

Baird, D. D. and Wilcox, A. J. (1985). Cigarette smoking associated with delayed conception. *Journal of the American Medical Association,* **253,** 2979–83.

Baird, D. D., Weinberg, C. R., and Rowland, A. (1991). Misclassification in time to pregnancy data: Impact on estimates of fecundability. *American Journal of Epidemiology,* **133,** 1282–90.

Baron, J. A. (1984). Smoking and estrogen-related dieases. *American Journal of Epidemiology,* **119,** 9–22.

Christianson, R. E., Oechsli, F. W., and Van Den Berg, B. J. (1989). Caffeinated beverages and decreased fertility. *Lancet,* **i,** 378.

Daling, J., Weiss, N., Spadoni, L., Moore, D. E., and Voigt, L. (1987). Cigarette smoking and primary tubal infertility. In *Smoking and reproductive health,* (ed. M. J. Rosenberg), pp. 40–6. PSG, Littleton, Massachusetts.

De Mouzon, J. Spira, A., and Schwartz, D. (1988). A prospective study of the relation between smoking and fertility. *International Journal of Epidemiology,* **17,** 378–84.

Friedman, S. (1977). Artificial donor insemination with frozen human semen. *Fertility and Sterility,* **28,** 1230–3.

Harlap, S. and Baras, M. (1984). Conception-waits in fertile women after stopping oral contraceptives. *International Journal of Fertility,* **29,** 73–80.

Hartz, A. J., Kelber, S., Borkowf, H., Wild, R., Gillis, B. L., and Rimm, A. A. (1987). The association of smoking with clinical indicators of altered sex steroids—a study of 50,145 women. *Public Health Reports,* **102,** 254–9.

Hatch, E. E. (1990). The association of delayed conception with cigarette smoking and caffeine intake. Doctoral Dissertation. Yale University, New Haven, Connecticut.

Hirsch, M. B. and Mosher, W. D. (1987). Characteristics of infertile women in the United States and their use of infertility services. *Fertility and Sterility*, **47**, 618–25.

Hogue, C. J. R. and Sappenfield, W. (1987). Smoking and low birth weight: current concepts. In *Smoking and reproductive health*, (ed. M. J. Rosenberg), pp. 97–102. PSG, Littleton, Massachusetts.

Howe, G., Westhoff, C., Vessey, M., and Yeates, D. (1985). Effects of age, cigarette smoking, and other factors on fertility: findings in a large prospective study. *British Medical Journal*, **290**, 1697–1700.

Hull, M. G., Glazener, C. M., Kelly, N. J., Conway, D. I., Foster, P. A., Hinton, R. A., *et al.* (1985). Population study of causes, treatment, and outcome of infertility. *British Medical Journal of Clinical Research*, **291**, 1693–7.

Joesoef, M. R., Beral, V., Rolfs, R. T., Aral, S. O., and Cramer, D. W. (1990). Are caffeinated beverages risk factors for delayed conception? *Lancet*, **i**, 136–7.

Linn, S., Schoenbaum, S. C., Monson, R. R., Rosner, B., and Ryan, K. J. (1982). Delay in conception for former 'pill' users. *Journal of the American Medical Association*, **247**, 629–32.

MacMahon, B., Trichopoulos, D., Cole, P., and Brown, J. (1982). Cigarette smoking and urinary estrogens. *New England Journal of Medicine*, **307**, 1063–5.

Mai, F. M., Munday, R. N., and Rump, E. E. (1972). Psychiatric interview comparisons between infertile and fertile couples. *Psychosomatic Medicine*, **34**, 431–40.

Mattison, D. R. (1982). The effects of smoking on fertility from gametogenesis to implantation. *Environmental Research*, **28**, 410–33.

Michnovicz, J. J., Hershcopf, R. J., Naganuma, H., Bradlow, H. L., and Fishman, J. (1986). Increased 2-hydroxylation of estradiol as a possible mechanism for the anti-estrogenic effect of cigarette smoking. *New England Journal of Medicine*, **315**, 1305–9.

Mosher, W. D. (1988). Fecundity and infertility in the United States. *American Journal of Public Health*, **78**, 181–2.

Mueller, B. A., Daling, J. R., Weiss, N. S., and Moore, D. E. (1990). Recreational drug use and the risk of primary infertility. *Epidemiology*, **1**, 195–200.

Olsen, J., Rachootin, P., Schiodt, A. V., and Damsbo, N. (1983). Tobacco use, alcohol consumption and infertility. *International Journal of Epidemiology*, **12**, 179–84.

Phipps, W. R., Albrecht, B., Cramer, D. W., Gibson, M., Schiff, I., Berger, M. J., *et al.* (1987). The association between smoking and female infertility as influenced by cause of the infertility. *Fertility and Sterility*, **48**, 377–82.

Rachootin, P. and Olsen, J. (1982). Prevalence and socioeconomic correlates of subfecundity and spontaneous abortion in Denmark. *International Journal of Epidemiology*, **11**, 245–9.

Rantala, M. L. and Koskimies, A. I. (1986). Infertility in women participating in a screening program for cervical cancer in Helsinki. *Acta Obstetricia et Gynecologica Scandinavica*, **65**, 823–5.

Rosenberg, M. J. (ed.) (1987). *Smoking and reproductive health*. PSG, Littleton, Massachusetts.

Rowland, A. S. (1989). The effects of nitrous oxide on the fecundability of dental assistants. Doctoral Dissertation. University of North Carolina, Chapel Hill, North Carolina.

Schreiber, G. B., Robins, M., Maffeo, C. E., Masters, M. N., Bond, A. P., and

Morganstein, D. (1988). Confounders contributing to the reported associations of coffee or caffeine with disease. *Preventive Medicine,* **17,** 295–309.

Sloss, E. M. and Frerichs, R. R. (1983). Smoking and menstrual disorders. *International Journal of Epidemiology,* **12,** 107–9.

Stillman, R. J., Rosenberg, M. J., and Sachs, B. P. (1986). Smoking and reproduction. *Fertility and Sterility,* **46,** 545–66.

Stubblefield, P. G., Monson, R. R., Schoenbaum, S. C., Wolfson, C. E., Cookson, D. J., and Ryan, K. J. (1984). Fertility after induced abortion: a prospective follow-up study. *Obstetrics and Gynecology,* **62,** 186–93.

Tokuhata, G. K. (1968). Smoking in relation to infertility and fetal loss. *Archives of Environmental Health,* **17,** 353–9.

Weinberg, C. R. (1990). Infertility and the use of illicit drugs. *Epidemiology,* **1,** 189–92.

Weller, R. H., Eberstein, I. W., and Bailey, M. (1987). Planning status of birth, prenatal care, and maternal smoking. In *Smoking and reproductive health*, (ed. M. J. Rosenberg), pp. 86–90. PSG, Littleton, Massachusetts.

Wentz, A. C. (1986). Cigarette smoking and infertility. *Fertility and Sterility,* **46,** 365–7.

Wilcox, A. J., Weinberg, C. R., and Baird, D. D. (1988). Caffeine beverages and decreased fertility. *Lancet,* **ii,** 1453–6.

Williams, M. A., Monson, R. R., Goldman, M. B., Mittendorf, R., and Ryan, K. J. (1990). Coffee and delayed conception. *Lancet,* **i,** 1603.

# 3. Ectopic pregnancy and smoking: confounding or causality?

*Oona Campbell*

## Introduction

Renewed interest in ectopic pregnancy began in the mid-1970s with observations of a marked increase in the rate of ectopic pregnancies (Beral 1975; Rubin *et al.* 1983). Around the same time, awareness of the reproductive consequences of smoking was growing and, by the early 1980s, reports of an association between smoking and ectopic pregnancy emerged.

The question posed in the title of this chapter—whether the association between ectopic pregnancy and smoking is a causal one or whether it is due to confounding by unmeasured variables—is one that frequently arises in relation to smoking. The argument for confounding runs as follows: smoking is a 'lifestyle' variable, an exposure associated with systematic differences, not just in smoking behaviour but in overall characteristics and 'lifestyle' of the smoker (Pederson and Stavraky 1987). Associations observed between smoking and adverse outcomes may be attributable to this 'lifestyle' rather than to smoking *per se*. A well known example where consensus has not been reached is the controversy over the role of smoking and potential confounding by sexual and reproductive behaviour in the aetiology of cervical cancer (Winkelstein *et al.* 1984; Clarke *et al.* 1985). In different circumstances, Yerushalmy (1971, 1972) and Hickey and colleagues (1978) argue that low birth weight is caused by attributes of the smoker rather than by smoking itself. Hickey *et al.* (1978) go further and claim that both smoking and low birth weight are 'symptoms of deficient maternal bioenergetic systems'.

The association between ectopic pregnancy and smoking has now been shown in several epidemiological studies (Matsunaga and Shiota 1980; Levin *et al.* 1982; Campbell 1983; WHO 1985; Thorburn *et al.* 1986*a, b*; Campbell and Gray 1987; Chow *et al.* 1988; Handler *et al.* 1989; Holt *et al.* 1989), but while much can be learned from well-designed epidemiological studies, it is unlikely that scepticism about the causal role of 'lifestyle' variables, such as smoking, will be overcome unless they are also backed by studies of the biological mechanisms. This is particularly the case when hypothesized confounders, such a pelvic inflammatory disease (PID), are difficult to measure (Fig. 3.1). Furthermore, there are unique reasons why the relationship between smoking and ectopic pregnancy needs special emphasis from both

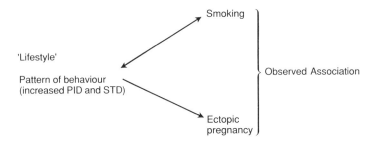

**Fig. 3.1.** Possible mechanism for confounding in the association between ectopic pregnancy and smoking.

epidemiological and laboratory researchers, if the issue, and the mechanism, of causality is to be resolved.

Epidemiological research on smoking and reproduction generally follows three lines of inquiry:

(1) does smoking impair couples'/women's fertility?
(2) does smoking lead to increased losses following conception?
(3) does smoking lead to adverse pregnancy outcomes?

Alternative lines of inquiry also examine the impact of smoking on subsequent outcomes in the infant, and on the reproductive system itself; these are beyond the scope of this discussion.

Broadly interpreted, any of these three lines of inquiry can encompass research on ectopic pregnancy. In practice, ectopic pregnancy is usually excluded from all three. The first question, for example, can be interpreted to consider the effect of smoking on the probability of ending up with a live birth (with ectopic pregnancy regarded as a failure to achieve this outcome). Most frequently, however, research in this field focuses on the effect of smoking on fecundability—the ability to conceive—and leaves out ectopic pregnancy, where the problem is not with conception but with the location of implantation. The second question, does smoking lead to increased losses following conception, is most widely interpreted as measuring the effect of smoking on the risk of spontaneous abortion, particularly in the absence of chromosomal defects. Finally, ectopic pregnancy can also be viewed as an adverse pregnancy outcome and included in the domain of the third question. Emphasis, however, is usually placed on late pregnancy outcomes such as birth weight, prematurity, and perinatal mortality (King and Fabro 1983; Cole 1986; Lincoln 1986; Stillman *et al.* 1986; Rosenberg 1987). As a result of this narrow conceptualization, it can be argued that general research on smoking and reproduction excludes, or fails to adequately consider, the issue of ectopic pregnancy.

In addition to difficulties stemming from the conceptualization of smoking and reproduction, three further characteristics of ectopic pregnancy contribute to its neglect within studies of smoking. Ectopic pregnancy is relatively rare compared to most other reproductive events under consideration, it is diagnosed at a comparatively early gestational age, and it has no suitable animal model.

The ectopic pregnancy rate is estimated at 1.4 per 100 pregnancies in the USA (1983) and 0.6 per 100 pregnancies in the UK (1982–4) (Chow *et al.* 1987; Turnbull *et al.* 1989). These rates are at least an order of magnitude lower than those of spontaneous abortion and low birth weight, the most commonly considered reproductive outcomes. Most studies designed to measure the impact of smoking on fecundability, spontaneous abortion, and adverse late pregnancy outcomes have sample sizes too small to demonstrate an impact on ectopic pregnancy.

The timing of ectopic pregnancy also makes it difficult to research within studies considering several outcomes. Ectopic pregnancy often becomes apparent at 6–8 weeks gestation and rarely fails to be identified by 10–12 weeks. Many prospective studies of pregnancy outcome on the other hand, recruit women some time into their pregnancy, often during their first antenatal care visit (Kullander and Kaellen 1971; Sandahl 1985). Sandahl (1985), for example, reports initiating follow-up at a mean of 17 weeks gestation, by which time ectopic pregnancies will have become apparent and women with this outcome will no longer be pregnant. Other prospective studies, which enrol women trying to conceive, have either failed to encounter ectopic pregnancy due to small sample sizes, or have failed to report and discuss it (Friedman 1977; Stubblefield *et al.* 1984; Howe *et al.* 1985; De Mouzon *et al.* 1988).

Finally, ectopic pregnancies are rare or unknown in animals. In rodents, ectopic pregnancy cannot be induced even when the uterotubal junction is occluded immediately following fertilization. Instead, the embryos degenerate after reaching the blastocyst stage (Speroff *et al.* 1989). Hodgen (1984) reports observing non-experimentally induced ectopic pregnancy only once in over 3000 non-human primate pregnancies. As no suitable animal models for ectopic pregnancy exist, researchers have to rely on epidemiological findings and on partial laboratory evidence from animals and humans.

For reasons implicit in the above discussion, evidence of the association between ectopic pregnancy and smoking did not emerge from general studies designed to assess the impact of smoking on reproduction. Rather, the association has primarily been demonstrated by case-control studies of ectopic pregnancy designed to measure other risk factors (Matsunaga and Shiota 1980; Levin *et al.* 1982; Campbell 1983; WHO 1985; Thorburn *et al.* 1986*a, b*; Campbell and Gray 1987; Chow *et al.* 1988; Handler *et al.* 1989; Holt *et al.* 1989). In several of these studies, smoking was not measured as part of a hypothesized relationship but rather as a potential confounder or measure of 'lifestyle' (Matsunaga and Shiota 1980; Levin *et al.* 1982; Campbell 1983; Gray 1985; WHO 1985; Thorburn *et al.* 1986*a, b*; Campbell and Gray 1987). Once attention was drawn to the association (Campbell and Gray

1987), subsequent studies assessed the plausibility of a causal relationship but only in terms of mechanisms that might elucidate their particular findings (Chow *et al.* 1988; Handler *et al.* 1989). This approach of *ex post facto* justification is adequate for initial findings but fails to consider fully the potential aetiological role of smoking in ectopic pregnancy. It is only by turning the issues on their head and developing a theoretical rationale for a causal smoking-ectopic association that the strengths and weaknesses of existing epidemiologic and laboratory evidence can be demonstrated.

## Aetiology of ectopic pregnancy

Ectopic pregnancy occurs when a conceptus implants outside the endometrium of the uterine cavity. Most ectopic pregnancies implant within the fallopian tube, with a small percentage sited in the abdominal cavity, the ovaries, the interstitium of the tube and uterus, and the cervix. In most cases the consequences of ectopic pregnancy are severe; the conceptus is invariably lost and the condition may be fatal to the mother (Droegemueller 1986).

In his review paper on smoking and fertility, Mattison (1982) outlines the multiple steps involved in reproduction:

Successful fertility results from the completion of a complex, stepwise process beginning with gametogenesis, continuing through gamete release, gamete interaction, conceptus transport, implantation, placentation, embryonic development, fetal growth and parturition.

In ectopic pregnancy, many of the steps take place, up to and including implantation and placentation. These last steps, however, do not occur in a site designed to receive the conceptus and permit it to develop. As a result of this inappropriate site of implantation, embryonic development, fetal growth, and parturition cannot occur in a normal manner.

Over the past 40 years, numerous predisposing conditions and biological mechanisms have been proposed to explain the occurrence of ectopic pregnancy. Frequently proposed mechanisms can be grouped under three major categories:

1. Conditions retarding or preventing the passage of the fertilized ovum into the uterus (including salpingitis and peritubal adhesions, developmental abnormalities, and tumours).
2. Conditions that increase tubal receptivity to the fertilized ovum (endometriosis).
3. Factors related to the gamete (including transmigration of the ovum, delayed ovulation, and abnormalities of the egg and/or sperm).

A common thread linking the most widely accepted of these aetiological theories is delay, especially delay in ovum transport. The following discussion of the possible aetiological role of smoking mainly addresses the issue of delay, elaborating on four potential contributors: delayed ovulation, altered motility, a combination of delayed ovulation and altered motility, and immunological alteration. Other aetiological possibilities with a potential role for smoking, including male factors (such as abnormal or low sperm count and abnormalities of the embryo), will not be discussed as there is no clear evidence that they are related to the occurrence of ectopic pregnancy (Droegemueller 1986; Chow *et al*. 1987). The possibility that the association between smoking and ectopic pregnancy is due to problems in study design or to confounding by unmeasured variables or 'lifestyle' is discussed in the consideration of the epidemiological evidence.

## Delayed ovulation

Iffy (1961) suggests that ectopic implantation may be caused by delayed ovulation, which in turn leads to late fertilization and inadequate development of the secretory endometrium. Menstruation occurs despite fertilization, and menstrual reflux—the backward washing of menstrual blood— flushes the conceptus back into the fallopian tubes or impedes its progress. Iffy proposed this mechanism to explain his finding that most ectopic embryos were 2 to 3 weeks older than menstrual data would indicate. More recently, ectopic pregnancy occurring during surrogate embryo transfer in monkeys has been interpreted as support for Iffy's theory (Hodgen 1984). Correspondence between Iffy (1984) and Hodgen (1984) argues that ectopic displacement and implantation due to retrograde lavage methods for collecting eggs and embryos mimics the effects of menstrual reflex.

A number of epidemiological and laboratory studies suggest one of the sites of action of smoking to be the hypothalamic–pituitary–ovarian axis (Mattison 1982; Stillman *et al*. 1986). This would allow smoking to exert an effect on the timing and nature of ovulation. Animal studies have demonstrated that nicotine or cigarette smoke influences this axis by altering the mechanisms controlling the release of gonadotropins and cyclicity (Stillman *et al*. 1986). Blake *et al*. (1972) demonstrated that, depending on the dosing schedule, subcutaneous injections of nicotine tartrate prior to and during the expected proestrous luteinizing hormone (LH) surge, delay and diminish, or inhibit the surge in sexually mature, cycling rats. Blake and colleagues also argue that the locus of this effect is outside the pituitary, as nicotine does not alter the pituitary's response to gonadotropin-releasing hormone (GnRH) or ether. Complementary work by McLean *et al*. (1977) investigates the acute effects of tobacco smoke inhalation prior to the expected LH surge on proestrous female rats. In their experiment, cigarette smoke delays, but does not blunt, the LH surge in a dose-dependent manner. Low nicotine cigarettes delay the surge by about 2 h while the high nicotine cigarettes delay it by about 5 h. The delay also reduces the number of rats ovulating, although McLean *et al*. argue that the levels of LH were sufficient to induce ovulation.

Winternitz and Quillen (1977) carried out a preliminary experimental study of acute hormonal responses to cigarette smoke. They failed to demonstrate changes in FSH or LH levels in women but had to abandon their study as the level of nicotine exposure used in their smoking protocol made their subjects ill (Mattison 1982). Finally, and more generally, epidemiological studies have suggested that female smokers have elevated levels of infertility, secondary amenorrhea, and menstrual abnormalities (Stillman *et al.* 1986; Mattison 1982).

Although the sum of these experiments and studies does not directly demonstrate an effect on the hypothalamic–pituitary–ovarian axis, it does suggest that acute exposure to nicotine or cigarette smoke diminishes LH, either directly or through its enhancement of vasopressin, and that its effects may be felt midcycle with the FSH and LH surges rather than in periods of tonic gonadotropin release. Studies of the effects of acute and chronic cigarette smoking on ovulation in women have not been identified in the literature although they should now be possible with urinary assay techniques.

## Altered motility

The most popular theories of the aetiology of ectopic pregnancy relate not to delayed ovulation but to delays of the ovum and conceptus in the fallopian tube. Delay is thought to arise either from altered motility or because infection leaves adherent mucosal folds that trap the ovum and/or alter its transport. Several studies suggest that smoking may play a role in altering motility by changing the pattern of spontaneous contractions in the fallopian tube, the uterofallopian junction and the uterus. Neri and Ekerling (1969) studied the effect of cigarette smoking on the patency of the fallopian tubes using a Rubin test and measured the tone and frequency of contraction of the uterotubal junction and the uterus. Fertile women in the follicular phase (days 8–12), who smoked fewer than four cigarettes per day, were tested in four groups: before and after smoking one cigarette; treatment with intramuscular adrenaline; treatment with intramuscular normal saline; and no treatment. The Rubin test showed that, compared to the period immediately prior to cigarette smoking, smoking significantly increased the uterotubal wave amplitude and tone. Results also showed that smoking increased the resting tone of the uterus and the amplitude of the uterine contractions, but not the frequency of contractions.

Neri and Marcus (1972) extended their work on women by studying the effects of nicotine on both the follicular and luteal phases of the Rhesus monkey. In the follicular phase, nicotine injections produced a biphasic effect with a brief increase in oviductal tone and contraction followed by a longer period of quiescence. During the luteal phase, nicotine treatment increased the frequency of tubal contractions but had little effect on tone or contraction amplitude. Similar responses were observed by Ruckebusch (1975) after exposure of rabbits to cigarette smoke.

MacMahon *et al.* (1982) report smokers as having significantly lower concentrations of urinary oestriol, oestradiol, and oestrone during the luteal phase of ovulatory cycles compared to non-smokers, although they found no differences in ovulation between the two groups. It is possible that these altered oestrogen–progesterone relationships may also affect tubal motility. There is also epidemiological evidence that pregnancies following administration of post-ovulatory oestrogens are a greater risk of being ectopic (Chow *et al.* 1987).

Although many gaps in information on the effects of smoking on tubal motility remain, the above-mentioned effects may translate into altered uterine and tubal function. In turn, altered motility may modify the length of time the conceptus remains in the fallopian tube by influencing the rate of contractions and conceptus transport and potentially lead to ectopic pregnancy.

Such mechanisms as altered conceptus transport are suggested by observations that nicotine delays implantation in the rat (Card and Mitchell 1976; Yoshinaga *et al.* 1979). In particular, Yoshinaga and colleagues studied the effect of pharmacological doses of nicotine on early pregnancy events in the rat. They were able to delay conceptus cleavage from the two-cell to four-cell stage, conceptus entry into the uterus, blastocyst formation, shedding of the zona pellucida, and implantation. Nicotine treatment was also found to change the spacing of the blastocysts and lead to crowding at the tubal end. Delayed implantation was not found to be due to low levels of circulating oestrogen as had been previously reported; rather nicotine-treated rats had oestrogen levels that were the same or higher than controls while progesterone levels were lower.

## Delayed ovulation and altered motility

A third possible mechanism consists of a combination of effects stemming from the possible impact of smoking on both delayed ovulation and altered motility. Evidence for each of these individual effects has been discussed in the previous sections. It is possible, however, that smoking simultaneously influences the LH and/or FSH surge in such a manner as to delay ovulation and the oestrogen–progesterone ratio to alter tubal motility. In this joint hypothesis, for which there is no independent experimental support, it is the cumulative delay of ovulation and reduced motility rather than menstrual reflux that leads to ectopic implantation.

## Immunological alterations

The final hypothesis ascribes delay due to abnormalities in tubal physiology arising from infection (Phipps *et al.* 1987). Cigarette smoking has been shown to adversely affect humoral and cell-mediated immunity in numerous studies (Onari *et al.* 1978, 1980; Hersey *et al.* 1983; Ginns *et al.* 1985). Such a reduction in immunity could affect the tubal epithelial responses to inflammation and result in an increased frequency of tubal infection and PID.

Supporting epidemiological evidence is presented by Mattison (1982) in his review of a small study by Drac and Kopecny (1970) showing that smokers are more likely to have vaginal infections with trichomonas, adnexal inflammation, and abnormal hysterosalpingograms. This finding could, however, be attributed to confounding by sexual behaviour. Data on fecundity in former smokers suggest that immunological pathways may not be very important in women, as impaired fecundity has not been observed in this group (Baird and Wilcox 1985; Daling et al. 1987; Phipps et al. 1987).

## Epidemiology

In light of the biological plausibility of a causal link between smoking and ectopic pregnancy, the next step is to consider the epidemiological evidence for an association. Despite the failure of studies of smoking and reproduction to hypothesize and consider possible effects on ectopic pregnancy, there are nevertheless several epidemiological studies with data on both smoking and ectopic pregnancy.

The increase in the rate of ectopic pregnancies noted in the mid-1970s instigated a number of hypotheses to account for the rise, including increases in the prevalence of IUD use, the practice of induced abortion, and the occurrence of sexually transmitted diseases (STD) leading to PID. These hypotheses sparked a number of studies, most of which used a case-control design. Seven of these provide data with which the smoking/ectopic pregnancy association can be examined, as summarized in Table 3.1. The results are abstracted in Table 3.2.

Attention was first drawn to the association between smoking and ectopic pregnancy with the presentation of results from a multinational World Health Organization (WHO) study (Campbell 1983; Gray 1985; WHO 1985; Campbell and Gray 1987). This matched case-control study observed a higher prevalence of current smoking among cases compared to both non-pregnant hospital controls and pregnant antenatal or abortion clinic controls. This increased prevalence among cases was observed in all 12 centres but the difference was greater in developing countries. After adjustment for other variables known or suspected to alter the risk of ectopic pregnancy (a history of PID or gonorrhoea, prior ectopic pregnancy, contraceptive method, tubal ligation, and induced abortion), current smoking was found to increase the risk significantly, except for the comparison with non-pregnant hospital controls in developed countries (Table 3.3). Interaction terms between smoking and other variables were included but were not significant and did not change the risk estimates markedly. Former smokers showed no increased risk. This study also found elevated risks after exclusion of women with exposures to any known risk factors, except for the comparison with the non-pregnant control in developed countries. A history of prior ectopic pregnancy was too rare to permit examination of smoking among women with two or more ectopic pregnancies but the distribution of ectopic implantation sites showed

**Table 3.1** Characteristics of studies with data on ectopic pregnancy and smoking

| Reference | Year | Number of cases | Number of controls | Source of cases | Source of controls | Measure of smoking | Potential confounders measured |
|---|---|---|---|---|---|---|---|
| Matsunaga and Shiota (1980) | 1962–1974 | 24 (49) | 2772 (3903) | Nishimura embryo collection | Induced abortion | Yes/no | Age, gravidity, pregnancy wastage, laparotomy, occupation, regular menses, contraception, alcohol |
| | | | 64 (82) | | Myomatous uteri | | |
| Levin *et al.* (1982) | 1976–1978 | 85 (176) | 498 (866) | Boston Hospital | Controls delivered on same day as ectopic | Yes/no | Race, religion, payment method, parity, prior miscarriage, ectopic, OC, IUD, pelvic surgery, gonorrhea, PID, D & C |

**Table 3.1** (*Continued*)

| Reference | Year | Number of cases | Number of controls | Source of cases | Source of controls | Measure of smoking | Potential confounders measured |
|---|---|---|---|---|---|---|---|
| Campbell and Gray (1987) | 1978–1980 | 1108 (1136) | 1108 (1136) 1108 (1136) | 927 developing country cases 181 developed country cases | 2 matched controls per case 1 non-pregnant hospital control 1 antenatal or abortion clinic control | Current, former, never; at time of interview | Age, race, centre, parity, date of admission, martial status, PID, gonorrhea, contraception, tubal ligation, induced abortion, prior ectopic |
| Thorburn *et al.* (1986a) | 1981–1982 | 205 (247) | 110 (11337) 101 (4605) | 5 hospitals in Gothenburg area | 3 hospitals Antenatal clinics Abortion clinics | Smoke ≤ 5 Smoke > 5 | Age, marital status, race, occupation, height, weight, infertility, planned pregnancy, regular menses, endometriosis, parity, miscarriage, induced abortion, D & C, PID, ectopic, abdominal |

| | | | | | | Smoking variables | | |
|---|---|---|---|---|---|---|---|---|
| Chow *et al.* (1988) | 1975–1979 | 155 (312) | 456 (607) | 5 King County hospitals | Vital statistics of live births. County residents (12 hospitals) | Current, former, never; age started; duration; no. per day; status at conception | surgery, hysterosalpingogram, medication, alcohol | Gravidity, race, Dalkon shield, condom, douching, year of pregnancy, income, occupation, number of marriages, number of partners, religion, education |
| Holt *et al.* (1989) | 1981–1986 | 221 (396) | 457 (1139) | Group health Co-op, Puget Sound | Co-op members at risk of pregnancy | Current, former, never; status at conception | | Race, religion, education, income, marital status, PID, IUD, parity, gravidity, spontaneous or induced abortion, age at first intercourse, number of partners |

**Table 3.1** (*Continued*)

| Reference | Year | Number of cases | Number of controls | Source of cases | Source of controls | Measure of smoking | Potential confounders measured |
|---|---|---|---|---|---|---|---|
| Handler *et al.* (1989) | 1983–1987 | 634 | 4287 | 12 hospitals, Univ Illinois Perinatal Network | 5% sample of live births in network | Yes/no; number per day | Race, age, payment method, gravidity, parity, prior miscarriage, induced abortion |

( ) under the number of cases and controls is the number originally identified while the number without parentheses is the actual number of cases or controls used. For example, Matsunaga and Shiota identified 49 cases but only used 24 in the smoking analysis. Where two numbers are shown, then two different types of control were used. For example, Matsunaga and Shiota used 2772 induced abortion controls and 64 myomatous uteri controls. OC, oral contraceptive; IUD, intrauterine device; PID, pelvic inflammatory disease; D & C, dilatation and curettage.

**Table 3.2** Association of smoking with ectopic pregnancy

| Studies | Odds ratio | Confidence limits | Type of control | Potential confounders controlled |
|---|---|---|---|---|
| Matsunaga and Shiota (1980) | 2.3 | 1.0–5.5 | Induced abortion | None |
| Levin *et al.* (1982) | 1.5 | 0.8–2.8 | Deliveries | Abortion, ectopic, PID, payment method, pelvic surgery, gonorrhoea, D & C, IUD, race, religion, parity, pill use |
| Campbell and Gray (1987) | 4.0 2.2 2.4 1.1 | 2.7–5.9 1.3–3.6 1.6–3.4 0.6–1.9 | LDC pregnant DC pregnant LDC hospital DC hospital | PID, gonorrhoea, ectopic, contraceptive method, sterilization, induced abortion, marital status, age, race, centre |
| Thorburn *et al.* (1986a) | 2.0 0.8 | | Antenatal Induced abortion | None |
| Chow *et al.* (1988) | 2.2 | 1.4–3.4 | Live births | Gravidity, race, Dalkon, condom, douche, year of pregnancy |
| Holt *et al.* (1989) | 1.6 | 1.0–2.5 | General population | None |
| Handler *et al.* (1989) | 2.3 | 1.9–2.7 | Live births | Race, age, spontaneous abortion |

LDC, less developed countries; DC, developed countries; PID, pelvic inflammatory disease; D & C, dilatation and curettage; IUD, intrauterine device.

a non-significant, though suggestive, increase in proximal implantation sites among smokers (12 per cent) compared with non-smokers (8 per cent) (Campbell and Gray 1987).

Two previous studies had also observed an association with smoking but judged it to have arisen through confounding. In a cross-sectional study, Matsunaga and Shiota (1980) explored the possibility that limited physical

**Table 3.3** Adjusted odds ratios for smoking as a risk factor for ectopic pregnancy: WHO multicentre case-control study

|  | Developing countries ($n = 927$) | Developed countries ($n = 181$) |
| --- | --- | --- |
| Pregnant controls |  |  |
| Adjusted smoking odds ratio | 4.0 | 2.2 |
| 95% confidence limits | (2.7–5.9) | (1.3–3.6) |
| Non-pregnant controls |  |  |
| Adjusted smoking odds ratio | 2.4 | 1.1 |
| 95% confidence limits | (1.6–3.4) | (0.6–1.9) |

Adapted from Campbell and Gray (1987)

space, due to ectopic implantation or enlarged myoma, caused localized malformations in the embryo. They found an excess of smokers among women with ectopic pregnancy compared to an induced abortion control (RR = 2.3; 95 per cent CL (confidence limits) = 1.0–5.5) but did not adjust for other risk factors. Levin *et al.* (1982) found that in their case-control study smoking was associated with an increased but non-significant risk of ectopic pregnancy (RR = 1.5; 95 per cent CL = 0.8–2.8) after adjustment for 15 variables, including induced abortion, prior ectopic pregnancy, PID, gonorrhoea, pelvic surgery, prior dilatation and curettage (D and C), payment method, and race. Both studies considered the smoking/ectopic association to have arisen through confounding or by chance and failed to discuss it in any detail.

Thorburn *et al.* (1986*a*) also report a higher prevalence of smoking among cases of ectopic pregnancy (42 per cent) compared to pregnant controls intending to continue gestation to term (26.4 per cent) but not to those seeking induced abortions (48.5 per cent). In a second publication, Thorburn *et al.* (1986*b*) fail to report results on smoking in their expanded analysis, presumably because it was no longer significant.

In contrast to earlier research, studies by Chow *et al.* (1988), Handler *et al.* (1989), and Holt *et al.* (1989) appear to have explicitly considered a smoking mechanism in their design. Chow *et al.* (1988) conducted a case-control study of tubal pregnancy using delivered women as the comparison group. They found a relative risk of 2.2 for current smokers (95 per cent CL = 1.4–3.4) and 1.6 for past smokers (95 per cent CL = 1.0–2.8) after adjusting for gravidity, race, vaginal douching, contraceptive method, and year of the reference pregnancy. Maternal age, religion, education, occupation, family income, hospital of treatment, history of abdominal or pelvic surgery, use of oral contraceptives, previous planning of the reference pregnancy, and use of coffee or alcohol were not included in the adjustment model as they made no appreciable difference. Similarly, number of sexual partners and age at first intercourse had no effect. No attempts at adjustment for PID or STD were made, despite the availability of this information, because Chow *et al.* argue that these may be part of the causal pathway acting indirectly through impaired immunity.

Chow *et al.* (1988) also failed to find much influence of other characteristics of a woman's smoking history (such as average number of cigarettes smoked per day, age at onset, duration, and pack years) on the size of the smoking risk. The failure to demonstrate a dose or a duration response, and the increased risk seen in former smokers, leads Chow and colleagues to argue against an 'acute' effect on ovum transport and for a hypothesis of reduced humoral and cellular immunity.

Handler and colleagues (1989) conducted a larger study using a perinatal registry to identify cases and controls. When ectopic cases are compared to controls delivered of a single live birth, a crude odds ratio of 2.3 (95 per cent CL = 1.9–2.7) is observed. Adjustment for maternal age, race, payment method, gravidity, parity, and spontaneous abortion separately does not alter the crude estimate (range 2.3–2.4), although a history of spontaneous abortion appears to interact with smoking. Among women without a prior history of spontaneous abortion, the odds ratio, adjusted for maternal age and race is 2.5 (95 per cent CL = 1.9–3.2). A significant dose gradient is seen with number of cigarettes smoked irrespective of whether this is expressed as a continuous ($p = 0.001$) or a categorical variable.

Finally, Holt and colleagues (1989) studied ectopic pregnancy by comparing ectopic cases to a group of randomly selected reproductive age women at risk of becoming pregnant. Information on current, former, and never smoking was collected and results presented suggest a higher prevalence of current smokers among cases as compared to controls (38.4 versus 28.4 per cent). Information is also available to adjust the crude odds ratio for a number of variables including PID, STD, and sexual history. Unfortunately Holt *et al.* have not reported these results to date.

The epidemiological evidence presented for an association between smoking and ectopic pregnancy has several limitations. The observed association may arise from confounding by unmeasured variables. Some studies failed (or were unable) to collect information on probable confounders relating to PID and STD (Matsunaga and Shiota 1980; Handler *et al.* 1989), and all studies except Chow *et al.* (1988) and Holt *et al.* (1989) failed to measure and control for sexual history. It is also possible that despite controlling for identified PID and STD, subclinical disease, which could not be measured, was also present and may have confounded the association between smoking and ectopic pregnancy. Alternatively, as smoking is a contraindication for certain methods of contraception, such as the pill, women smokers may be more

likely to be prescribed alternative methods of contraception, such as the IUD
or tubal ligation, which have a higher risk of ectopic pregnancy.

In addition to problems with confounding, many studies have also experienced problems in study design. Several (Matsunaga and Shiota 1980; Levin
*et al.* 1982; Thorburn *et al.* 1986*a*, *b*; Campbell and Gray 1987) have relied on
crude measures of smoking (yes/no; ≤ 5/>5 per day; current/former/never)
and most (except Chow *et al.* (1988) and Holt *et al.* (1989)) fail to ascertain
smoking at the time of conception and refer to smoking at the time of
interview instead. While it is likely that the majority of women display the
same smoking behaviour at conception and interview, confusion of the temporal sequence and misclassification may have occurred for some women.

Misclassification of the outcome variable may also have occurred: Chow *et
al.* (1988), Handler *et al.* (1989) and Holt *et al.* (1989) do not obtain histo-
pathological confirmation of ectopic pregnancy but use a presenting or discharge diagnosis instead. Missing observations on smoking status or further
subsetting of the cases or controls may also contribute to bias. In particular,
Matsunaga and Shiota (1980), Levin *et al.* (1982), Chow *et al.* (1987) and Holt
*et al.* (1989) exclude relatively large numbers of individuals (see Table 3.2).

Finally, potential biases arise from the choice of the control group, particularly as identification of an appropriate control is difficult for studies of
pregnancy outcome. Weiss *et al.* (1985) and Chow *et al.* (1987) recommend
using a general population sample of women at risk of pregnancy as controls,
yet all studies, except that of Holt *et al.* (1989) use pregnant controls, abortion
controls or hospital controls. The influence of these respective choices of
control can be seen in the WHO study (Campbell and Gray 1987) and the
Swedish study (Thorburn *et al.* 1986*a*) where two types of control were
selected (see Table 3.2). In both studies the risk relative to antenatal controls
was higher than the risk relative to abortion or hospital controls. For certain
outcomes, it is easy to speculate on the direction of the bias associated with an
inappropriate choice of control. For example, if smoking is a risk factor for
infertility and spontaneous abortion (Stillman *et al.* 1986), the use of a
pregnant control will elevate the risk associated with smoking, as pregnant
controls will have a deficit of smokers. The reverse may also be argued; in the
WHO study, for example, hospital controls were selected among non-
obstetric, non-gynaecological in-patients to avoid biases with respect to contraceptive use and PID. Patients in this group may have medical conditions
that are related to smoking habits and may underestimate the degree of
relationship.

An alternative way to resolve the question of possible confounding by PID
may be through aggregate level analyses. A preliminary look at ecological
data from the UK and US shows that increases in ectopic pregnancy are not
paralleled by similar increases in smoking. On the contrary, smoking rates
can be seen to decrease or remain constant while rates of ectopic pregnancy
and PID increase. However, tabulated data do not permit sufficient dis-
aggregation of the data to rule out an association.

# Conclusion

Laboratory research on humans and animals has provided adequate evidence for postulating a plausible biological effect of either acute or chronic smoking on ectopic pregnancy. Certain characteristics of the epidemiology of ectopic pregnancy have meant, however, that consideration of this particular outcome has been neglected in general studies of smoking and reproduction. Nevertheless, an association has been observed and many of the criteria for causality are present.

Epidemiological studies consistently show an increased risk of ectopic pregnancy among smokers. The magnitude of the estimate is usually around 2 but can range between 1.5 and 4.0. This elevated risk persists in those studies that attempt to adjust for suspected confounders and/or known risk factors, but few studies manage to collect information on sexual history. Furthermore, it is not possible to adjust for subclinical tubal infection or for certain aspects of sexual behaviour, and even restricting analysis to a subset without known risk factors does not eliminate this problem.

Information collected on cigarette smoking was limited in most studies and dose–response relationship could only be examined in two studies. Chow *et al.* (1988) fail to observe a dose–response relationship but this may be accounted for by their small sample size. Furthermore, it has been suggested that number of cigarettes smoked is not the best indicator of dose, as compensatory behaviour between the number of cigarettes smoked and the actual nicotine dose received is frequent. By contrast, the study of Handler *et al.* (1989), with a larger sample size, finds a significant dose–response effect. Poor measurement of smoking in many studies also means that smoking was measured after conception and implantation and requirements for temporal sequence are not always fulfilled. The WHO study (Campbell and Gray 1987) provides some data suggesting specificity of the smoking effect: a trend towards proximal implantation in smokers compared to non-smokers. Other studies have not reported such findings in their data.

In response to the question of confounding or causality, the evidence summarized above is strongly suggestive of a causal association between smoking and ectopic pregnancy but it does not exclude the possibility that the association is due to confounding or poor study design. It seems unlikely, however, that an epidemiological study that adequately measures and controls for PID can be designed in the near future. A hypothetical analysis of the level of association necessary for an unmeasured confounder to produce the observed effect may be conducted. This approach has been used by Winkelstein *et al.* (1984) with smoking and cervical cancer. In any case, one of the causal mechanisms may be an indirect effect acting through reduced immunity and PID, a mechanism favoured by Chow *et al.* (1988). Studies to date, with the exception of this latter study, do not support any particular causal mechanism. Not enough consistent evidence is available from former smokers to rule out either a chronic or an acute effect of smoking.

**Table 3.4** Percentage of adult female smokers in various countries

| Country | Sample | Year | Product | Percentage |
|---|---|---|---|---|
| Australia | National | 1983 | c | 30 |
| Canada | National | 1983 | c, ci, p | 32 |
| France | National | 1978 | c | 20 |
| Germany FDR | National | 1980 | c, ci, p | 29 |
| Ireland | National | 1980 | c, ci, p | 36 |
| Italy | National | 1981 | c | 32 |
| Japan | National | 1980 | c | 14 |
| New Zealand | National | 1981 | c | 29 |
| Norway | National | 1982 | c | 34 |
| Poland | National | 1980 | c, ci, p | 29 |
| Sweden | National | 1982 | c | 30 |
| UK | National | 1982 | c | 33 |
| USA | National | 1980 | c | 30 |
| Brazil | Sao Paulo | 1972 | c | 20 |
|  | workers | 1983 | c | 37 |
| China | Shanghai Co. | 1981 | c | 3 |
| Egypt | National | 1982 | c, p | 1 |
| Guatemala | Urban | 1972 | c | 10 |
| Hong Kong | National | 1984 | c | 4 |
| Indonesia | Various | 1984 | c | 10–15 |
| Israel | National | 1983 | c | 30 |
| Ivory Coast | Abidjan | 1981 | c | <1 |
| Kuwait | National | 1980 | c | 12 |
| Nepal | Urban | 1980 | b, p | 14 |
|  | Other | 1984 | b, p | 58–72 |
| Pakistan | Karachi | 1982 | c, b, p, ci | 6 |
| Papua New Guinea | Various | 1981 | c, local | 76–80 |
| Singapore | National | 1975 | c, ci, p | 8 |
| Thailand | Urban | 1981 | c | 4 |
|  | Rural | 1981 | c, local | 40 |
| Tunisia | Urban | 1984 | c, p | 6 |
| Zambia | Lusaka | 1984 | c | 56 |

c, cigarettes; ci, cigars, cheroots; p, pipe, hookah; b, bidi.
  Adapted from: Zaridze, D. G. and Peto, R. (ed.) (1986) *Tobacco: a major international health hazard.* IARC, Lyon.

Smoking is quite prevalent in developed countries; estimates in the 1980s for many countries in Europe and North America ranged between 30 and 35 per cent of adult women (Zaridze and Peto 1986). Furthermore, while women do quit smoking during pregnancy, many do so only after they are aware of the pregnancy, that is, after implantation (and the potential ectopic pregnancy) has occurred (Kleinman and Kopstein 1987). Although case fatality has been decreasing over the years, untreated ectopic pregnancies often result in maternal death and ectopic pregnancy remains one of the leading single causes of maternal mortality. Even after successful surgery, the prognosis for future fertility is poor and women are at a high risk of repeat ectopic pregnancy (Chow *et al.* 1987).

Finally, it is important to state that women in developing countries also smoke, and that the prevalence can be quite high. This figure rises sharply if local tobacco products are included or certain subgroups of the population are examined (Table 3.4). Even with a small attributable risk, considerable numbers of women in developing countries could suffer ectopic pregnancies, which, in the absence of accessible medical facilities and good diagnoses and treatment, expose women to extremely high risks of maternal mortality.

## Acknowledgements

I would like to acknowledge the support of Ronald Gray, who encouraged me to present this work. I am also indebted to Betty Kirkwood, who suggested numerous editorial and technical improvements to this paper, and to Lynne Davies who prepared the tables.

## References

Baird, D. D. and Wilcox, A. J. (1985). Cigarette smoking associated with delayed conception. *Journal of the American Medical Association*, **253**, 2979–83.

Beral, V. (1975). An epidemiological study of recent trends in ectopic pregnancy. *British Journal of Obstetrics and Gynaecology*, **82**, 775–82.

Blake, C. A., Scaramuzzi, R. J., Norman, R. L., Kanematsy, S., and Sawyer, C. H. (1972). Effect of nicotine on the proestrous ovulatory surge of LH in the rat. *Endocrinology*, **91**, 1253–8.

Campbell, O. M. R. (1983). Analysis of a case control study of ectopic pregnancy: examination of risk factors, control selection bias, and diagnostic validation. Unpublished ScM. Thesis. Johns Hopkins University.

Campbell, O. M. and Gray, R. H. (1987). Smoking and ectopic pregnancy: a multinational case-control study. In *Smoking and reproductive health*, (ed. M. J. Rosenberg), pp. 70–4. PSG, Littleton, Massachusetts.

Card, J. P. and Mitchell, J. A. (1976). *Nicotine induced alterations in implantation and decidualization in the rat*. The Ninth Annual Meeting of the Society for the Study of Reproduction, Abstract no. 104. Philadelphia.

Chow, W-H., Daling, J. R., Cates, W., and Greenberg, R. S. (1987). Epidemiology of ectopic pregnancy. *Epidemiologic Reviews*, **9**, 70–94.

Chow, W-H., Daling, J. R., Weiss, N. S., and Voigt, L. F. (1988). Maternal cigarette smoking and tubal pregnancy. *Obstetrics and Gynecology*, **71(2)**, 167–70.

Clarke, E. A., Hatcher, J., McKeown-Eyssen, G. E., and Lickrish, G. M. (1985). Cervical dysplasia: association with sexual behaviour, smoking, and oral contraceptive use? *American Journal of Obstetrics and Gynecology*, **151(5)**, 612–16.

Cole, H. (1986). Studying reproductive risks, smoking. *Journal of the American Medical Association*, **255(1)**, 22–3.

Daling, J. R., Weiss, N., Spadoni, L., Moore, D. E., and Voigt, L. (1987). Cigarette smoking and primary tubal infertility. In *Smoking and reproductive health*, (ed. M. J. Rosenberg), pp. 40–6. PSG, Littleton, Massachusetts.

De Mouzon, J., Spira, A., and Schwartz, D. (1988). A prospective study of the relation between smoking and fertility. *International Journal of Epidemiology*, **17(2)**, 378–84.

Drac, P. and Kopecny, J. (1970). Sterilität bei Raucherinnen und Nichtrancherinnen. *Zentralblad Gynekology*, **27**, 865–6.

Droegemueller, W. (1986). Ectopic pregnancy. In *Obstetrics and gynecology*, (5th edn), (ed. D. N. Danforth and J. R. Scott). J. B. Lippincott, Philadelphia.

Friedman, S. (1977). Artificial donor insemination with frozen human semen. *Fertility and Sterility*, **28**, 1230–3.

Ginns, L. C., Ryu, J. H., Rogol, P. R., Sprince, N. L., Oliver, L. C., and Larsson, C. J. (1985). Natural killer cell activity in cigarette smokers and asbestos workers. *American Review of Respiratory Diseases*, **131**, 831–4.

Gray, R. H. (1985). A case-control study of ectopic pregnancy in developed and developing countries. In *Intrauterine contraception: advances and future prospects*, (ed. G. I. Zatuchni, A. Goldsmith, and J. J. Sciarra), pp. 354–64. Harper and Row, Philadelphia.

Handler, A., Davis, F., Ferre, C., Yeko, T. (1989). The relationship of smoking and ectopic pregnancy. *American Journal of Public Health*, **79(9)**, 1239–42.

Hersey, P., Prendergast, D., and Edwards, A. (1983). Effects of cigarette smoking on the immune system. Follow-up studies in normal subjects after cessation of smoking. *Medical Journal of Australia*, **2**, 425–9.

Hickey, R. J., Clelland, R. C., Bowers, E. J. (1978). Maternal smoking, birthweight, infant death and the self-selection problem. *American Journal of Obstetrics and Gynecology*, **131**, 305.

Hodgen, G. D. (1984). Embryo transfer and ectopic pregnancy (reply to letter). *Journal of the American Medical Association*, **251(20)**, 2660.

Holt, V. L., Daling, J. R., Voigt, L. F., McKnight, B., Stergachis, A., Chu, J., and Weiss, N. S. (1989). Induced abortion and the risk of subsequent ectopic pregnancy. *American Journal of Public Health*, **79(9)**, 1234–8.

Howe, G., Westhoff, C., Vessey, M., Yeates, D. (1985). Effects of age, cigarette smoking, and other factors on fertility: findings in a large prospective study. *British Medical Journal*, **290**, 1697–700.

Iffy, L. (1961). Contribution to the aetiology of ectopic pregnancy. *Journal of Obstetrics and Gynaecology of the British Commonwealth*, **68**, 441–50.

Iffy, L. (1984). Embryo transfer and ectopic pregnancy (letter). *Journal of the American Medical Association*, **251(20)**, 2660.

King, J. C. and Fabro, S. (1983). Alcohol consumption and cigarette smoking: effect on pregnancy. *Clinical Obstetrics and Gynecology*, **26(2)**, 437–48.

Kleinman, J. C. and Kopstein, A. (1987). Smoking during pregnancy, 1967–80. *American Journal of Public Health*, **77(7)**, 823–5.

Kullander, S. and Kaellen, B. (1971). A prospective study of smoking and pregnancy. *Acta Obstetrica et Gynecologica Scandinavica*, **50**, 83–94.

Levin, A. A., Schoenbaum, S. C., Stubblefield, P. G., Zimicki, S., Monson, R. R., and Ryan, K. J. (1982). Ectopic pregnancy and prior induced abortion. *American Journal of Public Health*, **72(3)**, 253–6.

Lincoln, R. (1986). Smoking and reproduction. *International Family Planning Perspectives*, **12(1)**, 22–6.

MacMahon, B., Trichopoulos, D., Cole, P., and Brown, J. (1982). Cigarette smoking and urinary estrogens. *New England Journal of Medicine*, **307**, 1063–5.

Matsunaga, E. and Shiota, K. (1980). Ectopic pregnancy and myoma uteri: teratogenic effects and maternal characteristics. *Teratology*, **21**, 61–9.

Mattison, D. R. (1982). The effects of smoking on fertility from gametogenesis to implantation. *Environmental Research*, **28**, 410–33.

McLean, B. K., Rubel, A., and Nikitovitch-Winer, M. B. (1977). The differential effects of exposure to tobacco smoke on the secretion of luteinizing hormone and prolactin in the proestrous rat. *Endocrinology*, **100(6)**, 1566–70.

Neri, A. and Ekerling, B. (1969). Influence of smoking and adrenaline (epinephrine) on the uterotubal insufflation test (Rubin test). *Fertility and Sterility*, **20**, 818–28.

Neri, A. and Marcus, S. L. (1972). Effect of nicotine on the motility of the oviducts in the rhesus monkey: a preliminary report. *Journal of Reproductive Fertility*, **31**, 91–7.

Onari, K., Seyama, A., Inamizu, T., Kodomari, N., Takaishi, M., Norioka, N., Ikuta, T., Iwamoto, K., Sadamoto, K., Katsube, M., Yamakido, M., and Nishimoto, Y. (1978). Immunological study on cigarette smokers. Part i. Serum protein pattern in smokers. *Hiroshima Journal of Medical Science*, **27**, 113–18.

Onari, K., Sadamoto, K., Takaishi, M., Inamizu, T., Ikuta, T., Yorioka, N., Ishioka, S., Yamakido, M., and Nishimoto, Y. (1980). Immunological study on cigarette smokers. Part ii. Cell mediated immunity in cigarette smokers and the influence of the water-soluble fraction (WSF) of cigarette smoke on the immunity of mice. *Hiroshima Journal of Medical Science*, **29**, 29–34.

Pederson, L. L. and Stavraky, K. M. (1987). Relationship of smoking to lifestyle factors in women. *Women and Health*, **12(2)**, 47–66.

Phipps, W. R., Albrecht, B., Cramer, D. W., Gibson, M., Schiff, I., Berger, J., Belisle, S., Wilson, E., and Stillman, R. (1987). The association between smoking and female infertility as influenced by cause of the infertility. *Fertility and Sterility*, **48**, 377–82.

Rosenberg, M. J. (ed.) (1987). *Smoking and reproductive health*. PSG, Littleton, Massachusetts.

Rubin, G. L., Peterson, H. B., Dorfman, S. F., Layde, P. M., Mage, J. M., Ory, H. W., Cates, W. Jr. (1983). Ectopic pregnancy in the United States, 1970–1978. *Journal of the American Medical Association*, **249**, 1725–9.

Ruckebusch, Y. (1975). Relationship between electrical activity in oviducts and uterus of the rabbit in vivo. *Journal of Reproductive Medicine*, **25**, 293.

Sandahl, B. (1985). A prospective study of drug use, smoking and contraceptives during early pregnancy. *Acta Obstetrica et Gynecologica Scandinavica*, **64**, 381–6.

Speroff, L., Glass, R. H., and Kase, N. G. (1989). *Clinical gynecologic endocrinology and infertility*, (4th edn). Williams and Wilkins, Baltimore.

Stillman, R. J., Rosenberg, M. J., and Sachs, B. P. (1986). Smoking and reproduction. *Fertility and Sterility*, **46(4)**, 545–66.

Stubblefield, P. G., Monson, R. R., Schoenbaum, S. C., Wolfson, C. E., Cookson, D. J., Ryan, K. J. (1984). Fertility after induced abortion: a prospective follow-up study. *Obstetrics and Gynecology*, **63**, 186–93.

Thorburn, J., Berntsson, C., Philipson, M., and Lindbolm, B. (1986*a*). Background factors of ectopic pregnancy. I. Frequency distribution in a case-control study. *European Journal of Obstetrics, Gynecology, and Reproductive Biology*, **23(5–6)**, 321–31.

Thorburn, J., Philipson, M., and Lindbolm, B. (1986*b*). Background factors of ectopic pregnancy. II. Risk estimation by means of a logistic model. *European Journal of Obstetrics, Gynecology, and Reproductive Biology,* **23(5–6),** 333–40.

Turnbull, A., Tindall, V. R., Beard, R. W., Robson, G., Dawson, I. M. P., Cloake, E. P., Ashley, J. S. A., and Botting, B. (1989). *Report on confidential enquiries into maternal deaths in England and Wales 1982–1984.* Department of Health, Report on Health and Social Subjects, 34. HMSO, London.

Weiss, N. S., Daling, J. R., and Chow, W.-H. (1985). Control definition in case-control studies of ectopic pregnancy. *American Journal of Public Health,* **75,** 67–8.

Winkelstein, W. Jr., Shillitoe, E. J., Brand, R., and Johnson, K. K. (1984). Further comments on cancer of the uterine cervix, smoking and herpes virus infection. *American Journal of Epidemiology,* **119,** 1–8.

Winternitz, W. W. and Quillen, D. (1977). Acute hormonal response to cigarette smoking. *Journal of Clinical Pharmacology,* **17,** 389–97.

World Health Organization (WHO) (1985). Special programme of research, development and research training in human reproduction. Task force on intrauterine devices for fertility regulation (1985). A multinational case-control study of ectopic pregnancy. *Clinical Reproduction and Fertility,* **3(2),** 131–43.

Yerushalmy, J. (1971). The relationship of parents' cigarette smoking to outcome of pregnancy: implications as to the problem of inferring causation from observed associations. *American Journal of Epidemiology,* **93,** 443.

Yerushalmy, J. (1972). Infants with low birth weight born before their mothers started to smoke cigarettes. *American Journal of Obstetrics and Gynecology,* **112,** 227.

Yoshinaga, K., Rice, C., Krenn, J., and Pilot, R. L. (1979). Effects of nicotine on early pregnancy in the rat. *Biology of Reproduction,* **20,** 294–303.

Zaridze, D. G. and Peto, R. (1986). *Tobacco: a major international health hazard.* IARC, Lyon.

# 4. Effects of maternal tobacco smoke inhalation on early embryonic growth

*Mary J Seller, Kulwinder S Bnait, and Nigel J Cairns*

## Introduction

Maternal cigarette smoking in pregnancy is associated with two well recognized effects—an increase in pregnancy wastage and low birth weight babies (Butler *et al.* 1972). These phenomena are well researched and it is known there is an inverse relationship between the number of cigarettes smoked and the decrease in birth weight and reduced fetal survival (reviewed by Abel 1980). Further, if a woman changes her smoking behaviour before the fourth month of pregnancy, then her outcome at delivery is appropriate to her pattern of smoking in the second part of pregnancy (Butler *et al.* 1972).

There are also data which suggest that, overall, congenital malformations are not increased in frequency in women who smoke during pregnancy, although in some populations specific abnormalities might occur more often. Examples are cleft lip, cleft palate (Andrews and McGarry 1972; Saxen 1974; Ericson *et al.* 1979), congenital heart disease (Fedrick *et al.* 1971), and neural tube defects (Evans *et al.* 1979).

In the face of no real diminution in tobacco consumption, the Independent Scientific Committee on Smoking and Health (ISCSH) has urged the modification of tobacco products so that the yields of tar, nicotine, and carbon monoxide of cigarettes is reduced. This has taken place to some extent, and it would appear to have reduced the frequency of some of the smoking-related diseases. However, there is evidence that some people compensate for the reduction in cigarette nicotine content by increasing their intake (ISCSH 1988).

This chapter describes the first results of a programme to examine the effects of maternal inhalation of tobacco smoke on embryonic development in the mouse. Most animal work in the literature has involved injection of nicotine and its derivatives, a route that does not parallel the human situation. The particular objectives have been to compare the effects of a modified cigarette with an unmodified one, and to compare the response of two genetically distinct strains of mice. One of these strains, additionally, bears a mutation that predisposes it to a specific congenital malformation (neural tube defects), although, in the bulk of the work reported here (which involves early embryonic development) this has not been particularly relevant.

## Materials and methods

### Mice

Two strains of mice were used: C57BL/6J, and CBA, which also bore the mutant gene curly-tail (CBA-ct/ct) (Grüneberg 1954). These mice are referred to as 'curly-tail'. The autosomal recessive gene, curly-tail, produces neural tube defects (NTD), manifest as exencephaly, open spina bifida or a curly tail. The gene is partially penetrant and roughly 60 per cent of the mice manifest one of the following abnormalities: rarely exencephaly, open spina bifida (in about 20 per cent of cases), and, most commonly, a curly tail (Embury *et al.* 1979), caused by delayed closure of the posterior neuropore (Copp *et al.* 1982). The remainder of the mice, though bearing the gene, are phenotypically normal.

Both strains of mice were closed-colony random bred. Males and females of each strain, aged 8–12 weeks, were placed together overnight and the females examined for plugs each morning. The day a plug was observed was designated day 0 of pregnancy. All mice were allowed free access to food and water at all times.

### Exposure to tobacco smoke

Mice were placed in a British–American Tobacco–Mason Inhalation machine, which provided nose-only exposure to tobacco smoke. Sham-treated mice were placed in the machine charged with unlit cigarettes, and remained there for the same duration as the smoking animals.

Two types of cigarette were used: the first, referred to as 'higher tar', had a total particulate matter of $12.9 \pm 1.1$ mg/cigarette; the second, called 'lower tar', had a total particulate matter of $4.8 \pm 1.1$ mg/cigarette. In all experiments the puff volume was $35 \pm 0.5$ cm$^3$, and the puff duration was 2 s.

Several different exposure regimes and doses were used. These are described in the individual experiments below.

### Assessment of embryonic development

For the studies on early embryonic development, pregnant mice were killed by cervical dislocation on day 9 of gestation. The uterus was exposed and the number of resorptions and live embryos counted. Each embryo was dissected from its membranes under a low power Wild stereomicroscope and assessed for developmental stage according to three parameters:

(1) whether the embryo had 'turned';
(2) whether the anterior neuropore had closed;
(3) the number of somites.

Conventionally, somite number is the most reliable index of stage of development.

For studies towards the end of gestation the mice were killed on day 18, the dead embryos were blotted after removal from the amniotic sac, weighed on a Mettler analytical balance, examined for major external and internal congenital abnormalities, and sexed on the basis of the internal genitalia.

## Nicotine and carbon monoxide estimations in maternal blood

Within minutes of the final exposure to tobacco smoke on day 8 of gestation, the pregnant mouse was killed by cervical dislocation, the carotid artery severed, and the blood collected in a heparinized capillary tube. The carbon monoxide content was assayed using the method of Buchwald (1969). Nicotine assay was carried out by a method developed from those of Garriatt (1975) and Jacob *et al.* 1981 by one of the authors (KSB) and Dr N Dalton (Department of Paediatric Renal Research, Guy's Hospital, London). It involved a double extraction, the use of lignocaine as the internal standard, and subjection of the extract to gas chromatography and mass spectrometry. The nicotine content was determined from the nicotine:lignocaine ratio of ions detected by the mass spectrometer.

Results were analysed statistically using the *t*-test for independent samples, and differences between means were regarded as significant if $P < 0.05$.

## Experiments and results

The first two experiments were pilot experiments to determine whether the system was sensitive enough to detect deleterious effects of tobacco smoke and also that it was a suitable model for the human situation.

## Experiment 1: exposure of curly-tail mice to smoke from 12 higher or lower tar cigarettes once a day from day 0 to day 8 of pregnancy

Curly-tail mice were exposed to 12 higher or lower tar cigarettes for 20 min once a day from the day of conception (day 0) to day 8 of pregnancy, and were killed on day 9. In sham-treated mice, the postimplantation embryonic loss was 6.3 per cent (Table 4.1). Eighteen per cent of the live embryos had an open anterior neuropore, all had turned, and the mean somite number was 16.8. Embryos of mothers that had been exposed to the 12 higher tar cigarettes had a mean somite number of 13.5, 54 per cent had an open anterior neuropore and 23 per cent were unturned. The embryonic loss was 12.5 per cent of the total implantations. Exposure to 12 lower tar cigarettes over the same time period also resulted in an embryonic loss rate of 12.5 per cent, 56 per cent of embryos had open neuropores and 33 per cent of embryos remained unturned. The mean somite number was 14.2. The difference in somite number between the untreated mice and the treated groups was statistically

**Table 4.1**  Effect of exposure to twelve cigarettes once a day from day 0 to day 8

| Curly-tail mice | Sham-exposed controls | Higher tar cigarettes | Lower tar cigarettes |
|---|---|---|---|
| Number of litters | 8 | 8 | 8 |
| Number of live embryos (mean litter size) | 60 (7.5) | 56 (7.0) | 63 (7.9) |
| Number of resorptions | 4 | 8 | 9 |
| Embryonic loss (% of total implantations) | 6.3% | 12.5% | 12.5% |
| Open anterior neuropore (% of total embryos) | 11 (18%) | 30 (54%) | 35 (56%) |
| Unturned (% of total embryos) | 0 (0%) | 13 (23%) | 21 (33%) |
| Mean somite number | 16.8 | 13.5 | 14.2 |

significant (higher tar $P < 0.0001$; lower tar $P < 0.0006$), but there was no difference between higher and lower tar cigarettes ($P = 0.31$). Thus, both higher and lower tar cigarettes from conception and through the pre- and early postimplantation stages were associated with increased embryonic loss and retardation in embryonic development, of a roughly similar magnitude.

## Experiment 2: exposure of curly-tail mice to smoke from 12 lower tar cigarettes once a day from day 0 to day 17 of pregnancy

The effects of more prolonged exposure were studied by continuing the treatment once a day to 12 lower tar cigarettes from day 0 through pregnancy until day 17. The embryos were assessed on day 18 (Table 4.2). In sham-treated mice, the embryonic loss was 3.3 per cent, the mean embryonic weight was 1.0597 g and 55 per cent of the embryos had NTD. But following cigarette smoke exposure, the embryonic loss was 17.5 per cent, the mean embryonic weight was 0.9120 g, and 54 per cent of embryos had neural tube defects. No other congenital malformations were observed. Thus, with continued maternal cigarette smoke exposure through pregnancy, there was a five-fold increase in intra-uterine embryonic death and the live embryos weighed significantly less, on average 14 per cent less, than sham-exposed mice; this difference was statistically significant ($P < 0.0001$). However, the number with NTD was no different from sham-exposed mice. As the first experiment showed that cigarette smoke exposure retards the embryos by the time of neurulation, the fact that there is no increase in NTD in mature embryos shows that the embryos are able to complete the normal developmental processes successfully despite the retardation.

**Table 4.2** Effects of exposure to twelve lower tar cigarettes once a day from day 0 to day 17

| Curly-tail mice | Sham exposed | Lower tar cigarettes |
|---|---|---|
| Number of litters | 5 | 5 |
| Number of live embryos (mean litter size) | 29 (5.8) | 33 (6.6) |
| Number of resorptions | 1 | 7 |
| Embryonic loss (% of total implantations) | 3.3% | 17.5% |
| Mean embryo weight (g) | 1.0597 | 0.9120 |
| Number of live embryos with neural tube defects (%) | 16 (55%) | 18 (54%) |

These two pilot experiments demonstrated the validity of the system. Daily maternal exposure to tobacco smoke through pregnancy resulted in the near-term embryos displaying the major phenomena observed in humans, namely low birth weight and increased pregnancy wastage. In addition, it was found that embryonic death and growth retardation were manifest as early as the neurulation stage of embryonic development with this daily exposure from conception. However, with this dose level no increase in a specific congenital malformation—neural tube defects—to which these mice are genetically predisposed, or any other malformation, was found.

## Experiment 3: exposure of two different strains of pregnant mice to smoke from six higher tar or lower tar cigarettes three times a day on days 6, 7, and 8

C57BL and curly-tail mice were exposed to six higher tar or six lower tar cigarettes for 10 min, three times a day, at 2.5-h intervals, on days 6, 7, and 8 of gestation. They were killed on the morning of day 9.

In sham-exposed C57BL mice the embryonic loss rate was 8.9 per cent, the mean somite number of live embryos was 18.06, the anterior neuropore was open in 2 per cent, and 1 per cent were unturned (Table 4.3). Exposure to higher tar cigarette smoke resulted in an embryonic loss of 31 per cent. The mean somite number was only 14.18 ($P < 0.0001$) and 17.9 per cent of the embryos had open anterior neuropores and 1 per cent were unturned. Exposure to lower tar cigarette smoke was associated with an embryonic loss rate of 23.4 per cent, a mean somite number of 14.94 ($P < 0.0001$), open anterior neuropores in 22 per cent of embryos, and 5 per cent of embryos remained unturned. The difference in somite number between higher tar and lower tar cigarette treatment was significant ($P = 0.027$).

**Table 4.3** C57BL mice: effect of exposure to six cigarettes three times a day on days 6, 7, and 8

| C57BL mice | Sham-exposed controls | Higher tar cigarettes | Lower tar cigarettes |
|---|---|---|---|
| Number of litters | 15 | 15 | 15 |
| Number of live embryos (mean litter size) | 122 (8.1) | 95 (6.3) | 108 (7.2) |
| Number of resorptions | 12 | 43 | 33 |
| Embryonic loss (% of total implantations) | 8.9% | 31.1% | 23.4% |
| Open anterior neuropore (% of total embryos) | 3 (2.5%) | 17 (17.9%) | 24 (22.2%) |
| Unturned (% of total embryos) | 1 (0.8%) | 1 (1.1%) | 6 (5.6%) |
| Mean somite number | 18.06 | 14.18 | 14.94 |

Thus, exposure of C57BL mice to the cigarette smoke over a 3-day period covering the immediate post-implantation phase of the embryos resulted in an increase in embryo lethality and a retardation in embryonic growth, and this was more noticeable in the higher tar than the lower tar group.

Sham-exposed curly-tail mice on the morning of day 9 had an embryonic loss rate of 8.2 per cent (Table 4.4), which was similar to that of C57BL mice,

**Table 4.4** Curly-tail mice: effect of exposure to six cigarettes three times a day on days 6, 7, and 8

| Curly-tail mice | Sham-exposed controls | Higher tar cigarettes | Lower tar cigarettes |
|---|---|---|---|
| Number of litters | 15 | 15 | 15 |
| Number of live embryos (mean litter size) | 100 (6.7) | 86 (5.7) | 85 (5.7) |
| Number of resorptions | 9 | 28 | 28 |
| Embryonic loss (% of total implantations) | 8.2% | 24.6% | 24.7% |
| Open anterior neuropore (% of total embryos) | 16 (16%) | 59 (68%) | 49 (58%) |
| Unturned (% of total embryos) | 4 (4%) | 29 (34%) | 16 (19%) |
| Mean somite number | 16.11 | 11.55 | 12.78 |

but the live embryos were less advanced developmentally, as their mean somite number was only 16.11 (the difference between the two strains being statistically significant: $P < 0.0001$), and 16 per cent still had open anterior neuropores. A small proportion (4 per cent) were unturned. Exposure to higher tar cigarettes resulted in 24.6 per cent embryonic loss, a mean somite number of only 11.5 ($P < 0.0001$), 68 per cent of embryos with open anterior neuropores and 34 per cent of embryos unturned. Following exposure to lower tar cigarettes, the embryonic loss was similar (25 per cent), the embryos were growth retarded, but less so than with the higher tar cigarettes—the mean somite number was 13.08 ($P < 0.0001$), 59 per cent had open anterior neuropores and 19 per cent were unturned. The difference in somite number between higher tar and lower tar cigarette treated embryos was significant ($P = 0.041$).

In comparing the responses of the two different mouse strains to the same tobacco smoke exposure, it must be remembered that an inherent difference between the two in the normal rates of early embryonic development has been observed; curly-tail mice are growing slightly more slowly than C57BL, having two somites less by the morning of day 9. They do, however, show similar rates of naturally occurring embryonic loss. Nevertheless, both strains show the same overall response to exposure to tobacco smoke on days 6, 7, and 8 of gestation, namely growth retardation and embryonic death, but in the curly-tail mice there is clearer evidence than in C57BL for the higher tar cigarettes having a greater detrimental effect on growth rate than the lower tar cigarette smoke—they are 4.61 somites behind the sham-treated embryos with higher tar, but only 3.03 somites behind with lower tar cigarettes. In addition, as the C57BL mice are only 3.88 somites behind after treatment with higher tar cigarette smoke, there is a suggestion that there might be a strain difference in response, with the curly-tail mice being more markedly affected than the C57BL mice. However, this difference could be related to the inherent differences in rate of development.

It is possible that the six cigarettes used in this experiment gave too high a dose, which tended to produce saturation, so masking some more subtle differential effects between the higher and lower tar types and between the two strains of mice. So the dose level was reduced to two cigarettes.

## Experiment 4: exposure of two different strains of pregnant mice to smoke from two higher tar or lower tar cigarettes, three times a day on days 6, 7, and 8

C57BL and curly-tail mice were exposed to two higher tar or two lower tar cigarettes for 10 min, three times a day, at 2.5-h intervals on days 6, 7, and 8 of pregnancy. In C57BL mice (Table 4.5) there was no increase in embryo mortality with maternal exposure to smoke from either two higher tar or two lower tar cigarettes. So a dose of two cigarettes, regardless of tar content, is

**Table 4.5** C57BL mice: effect of exposure to two cigarettes three times a day on days 6, 7, and 8

| C57BL mice | Sham-exposed controls | Higher tar cigarettes | Lower tar cigarettes |
|---|---|---|---|
| Number of litters | 15 | 15 | 15 |
| Number of live embryos (mean litter size) | 122 (8.1) | 122 (8.1) | 125 (8.3) |
| Number of resorptions | 12 | 14 | 6 |
| Embryonic loss (% of total implantations) | 8.9% | 10.3% | 4.6% |
| Open anterior neuropore (% of total embryos) | 3 (2.5%) | 17 (13.9%) | 6 (4.8%) |
| Unturned (% of total embryos) | 1 (0.8%) | 2 (1.6%) | 5 (4.0%) |
| Mean somite number | 18.06 | 16.46 | 17.60 |

not lethal to C57BL embryos. It does, however, still retard embryonic growth to some extent, but less so than with six cigarettes. The retardation is more marked with the higher tar cigarettes, where the somite number was 16.46 (compared with 18.06 in the controls; $P < 0.0001$), while lower tar cigarette smoke treated mice had 17.6 somites, which was not statistically different from the sham-treated ($P = 0.14$). There were similar findings with the other parameters of developmental rate.

In curly-tail mice, there was a clearer distinction between the response to higher and lower tar cigarettes (Table 4.6). Maternal exposure to the former doubled the embryonic mortality, while exposure to the latter had no effect on embryonic survival. Higher tar cigarettes produced significant embryonic growth retardation, the mean somite number being 12.92 ($P < 0.0001$)—that is, they were 3.14 somites behind controls, while similarly treated C57BL mice were only 1.6 somites behind—and 53 per cent of the embryos had open anterior neuropores and 21 per cent were unturned. By contrast, exposure of curly-tail mice to lower tar cigarette smoke produced a very similar, minor, degree of growth retardation as in the C57BL mice, with a mean somite number of 15.64, which was also not statistically significantly different from sham-treated embryos ($P = 0.25$). They were 0.47 of a somite behind control embryos while C57BL mice were 0.46 of a somite behind.

Thus, at this dose level, the curly-tail mice show a markedly different response to higher and lower tar cigarette smoke. Further, a differential response between two genetically different strains of mice has been demonstrated with respect to the higher tar cigarettes. Curly-tail mice are more susceptible to the effects of the higher tar tobacco smoke than C57BL mice,

**Table 4.6** Curly-tail mice: effect of exposure to two cigarettes three times a day on days 6, 7, and 8

| Curly-tail mice | Sham exposed controls | Higher tar cigarettes | Lower tar cigarettes |
|---|---|---|---|
| Number of litters | 15 | 15 | 15 |
| Number of live embryos (mean litter size) | 100 (6.7) | 90 (6.0) | 103 (6.9) |
| Number of resorptions | 9 | 19 | 11 |
| Embryonic loss (% of total implantations) | 8.3% | 17.4% | 9.7% |
| Open anterior neuropore (% of total embryos) | 16 (16%) | 48 (53%) | 26 (25%) |
| Unturned (% of total embryos) | 4 (4%) | 19 (21%) | 5 (5%) |
| Mean somite number | 16.11 | 12.92 | 15.64 |

as manifest by embryo lethality, which did not occur in the C57BL mice, and embryonic growth rate.

In addition, this entire set of experiments has demonstrated a clear dose response in both strains of mice. There is a greater effect on embryonic survival and growth rate with six cigarettes, than two cigarettes ($P < 0.001$ in all cases, except curly-tail, six higher tar versus two higher tar, where $P = 0.019$). This suggests the observations could be related to some of the components of tobacco smoke. Consequently, the next experiments examined the nicotine and carbon monoxide levels in the blood of the pregnant mouse following cigarette smoke exposure.

## Experiment 5: maternal blood nicotine levels following tobacco smoke exposure three times a day on days 6, 7, and 8 of gestation

Maternal blood was assayed immediately after the third exposure on day 8 of pregnancy. The sensitivity of the assay for nicotine has a lower limit of sensitivity of around 2 ng/ml. The assay registered a background amount of nicotine outside this range in sham-treated animals (Table 4.7), against which the levels in cigarette smoke exposed mice must be interpreted. There was a clear dose effect observed in both strains of mice. Smoke from six cigarettes produced higher levels of blood nicotine than two cigarettes, and higher tar cigarettes resulted in greater blood nicotine levels than lower tar cigarettes. With a dose of six higher tar cigarettes there was tendency for curly-tail mice to have higher nicotine levels than C57BL (mean values of 22.2 ng/ml, against 18.7 ng/ml), although there is some overlap, and the difference is not signi-

**Table 4.7** Mean blood nicotine levels on day 8 (treatment three times daily on days 6, 7, and 8)

| | Blood nicotine (ng/ml)* | | |
| --- | --- | --- | --- |
| | Sham exposed | Higher tar | Lower tar |
| 6 cigarettes | | | |
| C57BL | 0.24 ± 0.53 | 18.68 ± 8.76 | 13.26 ± 9.26 |
| Curly-tail | 0.22 ± 0.49 | 22.24 ± 6.47 | 12.66 ± 6.41 |
| 2 cigarettes | | | |
| C57BL | 0.24 ± 0.53 | 3.98 ± 2.01 | 0.04 ± 0.09 |
| Curly-tail | 0.22 ± 0.49 | 7.78 ± 0.98 | 1.78 ± 3.06 |

* Five mice in each group.

ficant ($P = 0.49$), while with six lower tar cigarettes the two strains have similar values—around 13 ng/ml ($P = 0.91$). With a dose of two higher tar cigarettes, however, the difference between the two strains was significant— curly-tail 7.8 ng/ml; C57BL 4.0 ng/ml ($P = 0.013$). This suggests that curly-tail mice absorb slightly more nicotine into the body than C57BL mice. This difference may be genetically determined. It is noteworthy that there was very little measurable nicotine in the blood of either C57BL or curly-tail mice after exposure to two lower tar cigarettes, although curly-tail mice, unlike C57BL, appeared to have a trace present.

## Experiment 6: maternal blood carboxyhaemoglobin levels following tobacco smoke exposure, three times a day on days 6, 7, and 8 of gestation

Maternal blood carboxyhaemoglobin (COHb) levels were estimated immediately after the third exposure on day 8. In sham-exposed mice some COHb was apparently measurable (Table 4.8). This reflects the limitations of the assay and represents a background against which the tobacco smoke exposed mice should be interpreted.

As with nicotine, a distinct dose response was observed in both strains of mice, both with respect to six cigarettes against two cigarettes, and higher tar and lower tar cigarettes. Exposure to smoke from six higher tar cigarettes produced significant levels of COHb in C57BL and curly-tail mice (21 and 22 per cent, respectively) while six lower tar cigarettes produced levels roughly half this amount (10.3 and 10.6 per cent, respectively). With two higher tar cigarettes, the tendency, noted with nicotine, for curly-tail mice to have higher levels than C57BL mice was also clearly present in the COHb levels (8.7 against 6.1 per cent; $P = 0.042$). It should be noted that whilst virtually

**Table 4.8** Mean blood carboxyhaemoglobin levels on day 8 (treatment three times daily on days 6, 7, and 8)

| | Blood carboxyhaemoglobin (%)* | | |
| --- | --- | --- | --- |
| | Sham exposed | Higher tar | Lower tar |
| 6 cigarettes | | | |
| C57BL | $0.9 \pm 0.6$ | $21.3 \pm 4.7$ | $10.3 \pm 2.1$ |
| Curly-tail | $1.3 \pm 0.6$ | $22.4 \pm 3.9$ | $10.6 \pm 2.3$ |
| 2 cigarettes | | | |
| C57BL | $0.9 \pm 0.6$ | $6.1 \pm 1.1$ | $2.1 \pm 1.5$ |
| Curly-tail | $1.3 \pm 0.6$ | $8.7 \pm 1.6$ | $2.8 \pm 1.8$ |

* Five mice in each group

no nicotine could be detected in the blood of either strain after exposure to two lower tar cigarettes, carboxyhaemoglobin was present, albeit in small amounts (C57BL 2.1 per cent; curly-tail 2.8 per cent).

## Correlation of the maternal blood levels of nicotine and carboxyhaemoglobin with the observations on embryos

The major findings have been summarized and correlated in Table 4.9.

Inhalation of tobacco smoke from a dose of six cigarettes, whether of higher tar or lower tar type, was associated with a marked increase in embryo lethality and embryo growth retardation, and significant levels of both nicotine and carboxyhaemoglobin were detected in the mother's blood. Despite the fact that six higher tar cigarettes produced both nicotine and COHb levels that were twice as high as those produced by six lower tar cigarettes, the effects on embryo lethality and growth rate produced by six higher tar cigarettes were not double those produced with six lower tar cigarettes; the difference was much less. With six higher tar cigarettes the pregnancy wastage was increased 3–3.5-fold over untreated animals, while with six lower tar cigarettes it was increased 2.5–3-fold, and the reduction in number of somites was 3.9–4.6 and 3.0–3.1, respectively. Interestingly, and possibly of significance, the effects of two higher tar cigarettes on curly-tail mouse embryo lethality (2-fold increase) and growth retardation (decrease of 3.2 somites) were broadly similar to the findings with six lower tar cigarettes in both strains, and the COHb levels were similar, at 8.7 per cent (curly-tail, two higher tar) as against 10.6 per cent (curly-tail, six lower tar; $P = 0.22$) and 10.3 per cent (C57BL six lower tar; $P = 0.17$), although the nicotine levels were less, at 7.8 ng/ml as against around 13 ng/ml in both cases ($P = 0.0009$ and $P = 0.0007$).

**Table 4.9** Summary and combination of all results

| | Higher tar | | Lower tar | |
|---|---|---|---|---|
| | C57BL | Curly-tail | C57BL | Curly-tail |
| **6 cigarettes** | | | | |
| Pregnancy wastage | ↑ × 3.5 | ↑ × 3.0 | ↑ × 2.6 | ↑ × 3.1 |
| Embryonic growth rate as measured by somite number | ↓ − 3.9 | ↓ − 4.6 | ↓ − 3.1 | ↓ − 3.0 |
| Nicotine levels (ng/ml) | 19 | 22 | 13 | 13 |
| Carboxyhaemoglobin levels (%) | 21 | 22 | 10 | 11 |
| **2 cigarettes** | | | | |
| Pregnancy wastage | No change | ↑ × 2.0 | No change | No change |
| Embryonic growth rate as measured by somite number | ↓ − 1.6 | ↓ − 3.2 | ↓ − 0.5 | ↓ − 0.5 |
| Nicotine levels (ng/ml) | 4 | 8 | 0 | 2 |
| Carboxyhaemoglobin levels (%) | 6 | 9 | 2 | 3 |

This suggests that there may be a relationship between a particular blood level of COHb and the degree of effect on the conceptus. The C57BL mice, by contrast, do not illustrate this point.

Looked at another way, the influence of particular blood levels of nicotine and COHb can be observed in mice treated with two cigarettes. In curly-tail mice, 8 ng/ml of nicotine and 9 per cent of COHb in the mother's blood are sufficient to double the pregnancy wastage and retard embryonic growth by as much as 3.2 somites. But 4 ng/ml of nicotine and 6 per cent COHb in C57BL mice did not produce any increase in embryonic death and retarded embryonic growth by only 1.6 somites.

The results with two lower tar cigarettes in C57BL mice are especially interesting because embryonic growth retardation is observed, albeit minimally (0.5 somites behind normal development), but this occurs in the face of negligible nicotine in the mother's blood, but still measurable COHb, suggesting that carbon monoxide and nicotine, separately, influence the embryonic growth rate.

## Confounding factors

To determine to what extent, if any, the results might be attributable to confounding factors such as a depression of the mother's appetite, which is known to occur with exposure to tobacco smoke, rather than to the tobacco products themselves, maternal body weight was examined.

## Experiment 7: maternal body weight before and after exposure to tobacco smoke exposure three times a day on days 6, 7, and 8 of pregnancy

The mice were weighed before the initial exposure to tobacco smoke on day 6, and then after the final exposure on day 8 (Table 4.10).

C57BL sham-treated mice tended to lose weight during the experimental period: however, not all did so—33 per cent gained weight. Thirty-eight per cent of the sham-treated curly-tail mice lost weight during the experiment, but the mean weight at the end of the experimental period represented an overall small weight gain. In both C57BL and curly-tail mice exposure to any of the smoking regimes resulted in weight loss, which was significantly different from the sham-treated mice, although three individual mice in different groups did exhibit a weight gain. In both types of mice, the extent of the weight loss was similar regardless of cigarette dosage, there being no significant difference between the treatment groups.

It is concluded that the recognized appetite-suppressing effect of exposure to tobacco smoke was manifest to some extent in the experiments, and could possibly be a factor in the growth retardation observed in the embryos. However, as the findings in the embryos demonstrated a marked dosage effect, but the maternal weight loss did not, maternal appetite suppression does not account for the findings in the embryos.

## Discussion

The main findings and some of their implications have already been discussed.

**Table 4.10** Maternal weight loss on day 8 (treatment three times daily on days 6, 7, and 8)

| Treatment | Weight loss (g) | | | |
|---|---|---|---|---|
| | C57BL | | Curly-tail | |
| | *n* | Mean (±SD) | *n* | Mean (±SD) |
| Sham exposed | 24 | 0.23 (0.67) | 13 | −0.03* (0.77) |
| 2 cigarettes lower tar | 11 | 1.04 (0.49) | 4 | 1.23 (0.79) |
| 6 cigarettes lower tar | 19 | 1.26 (0.49) | 16 | 0.89 (0.36) |
| 6 cigarettes higher tar | 30 | 1.17 (0.59) | 18 | 1.06 (0.54) |

* A negative value means that there was an overall weight gain.

With a standard intake of tobacco smoke, fixed as far as is possible by the smoking machine, marked differences in blood levels of nicotine and COHb are manifest with the two types of cigarettes, so the potential hoped for by modifying cigarettes to reduce yields of noxa is realized in the biological system presented in this paper. Overall, it has been found that the lower tar cigarette has a less detrimental effect on the conceptus than a cigarette with a higher tar content. However, if the dose of lower tar cigarette is high enough, the benefits are lost and the effects can be as severe as with the higher tar ones.

Evidence has been found for a slight difference in response between the two genetically different types of mice used in the effects on the conceptus of maternal exposure to tobacco smoke. This could be related to genetic differences in the speed of early embryonic growth, but another explanation could be that one strain actually takes more nicotine and carbon monoxide into the mother's blood. This itself could be genetically determined. The finding of a differential response between the two strains could have human parallels, with some women and/or their embryos being genetically predisposed to a greater or lesser response to tobacco smoke and its active constituents, and so explain the fact that not all women who smoke in pregnancy have small babies.

No evidence has been obtained (or sought in these experiments) as to the mechanisms by which the pregnancy wastage and embryonic growth retardation observed are mediated.

## Acknowledgements

This work was supported by the Tobacco Products Research Trust.

NJC was responsible for setting up and commissioning the smoking machine and performing experiments 1 and 2. KSB performed all the other work described.

## References

Abel, E. L. (1980). A review of effects on growth and development of offspring. *Human Biology,* **52,** 593–629.

Andrews, J. and McGarry, J. M. (1972). A community study of smoking in pregnancy. *Journal of Obstetrics and Gynaecology,* **79,** 1057–73.

Butler, N. R., Goldstein, H., and Ross, E. M. (1972). Cigarette smoking in pregnancy: its influence on birth weight and perinatal mortality. *British Medical Journal,* **2,** 127–30.

Buchwald, H. (1969). A rapid and sensitive method for estimating carbon monoxide in blood and its application in problem areas. *American Industrial Hygiene Association Journal,* **30,** 564–9.

Copp, A. J., Seller, M. J., and Polani, P. E. (1982). Neural tube development in mutant (curly tail) and normal mouse embryos: the timing of posterior neuropore closure in vivo and in vitro. *Journal of Embryology and Experimental Morphology,* **69,** 151–67.

Embury, S., Seller, M. J., Adinolfi, M., and Polani, P. E. (1979). Neural tube defects in curly-tail mice. I. Incidence, expression and similarity to the human condition. *Proceedings of the Royal Society of London. Series B,* **206,** 85–94.

Ericson, A., Kallen, B., and Westerholm P. (1979). Cigarette smoking as an etiologic factor in cleft lip and palate. *American Journal of Obstetrics and Gynecology,* **135,** 348–51.

Evans, D. R., Newcombe, R. G., and Campbell, H. (1979). Maternal smoking habits and congenital malformations: population study. *British Medical Journal,* **2,** 171–3.

Fedrick, J., Alberman, E. D., and Goldstein, H. (1971). Possible teratogenic effect of cigarette smoking. *Nature,* **231,** 529–39.

Garriatt, J. C. (1975). Type C procedure. In *Methodology for analytical toxicology,* (ed. I. Sunshine), pp. 121–3. CRC Press, Boca Raton, Florida.

Grüneberg, H. (1954). Genetical studies on the skeleton of the mouse. VIII. Curly-tail. *Journal of Genetics,* **52,** 52–67.

Independent Scientific Committee on Smoking and Health (ISCSH) (1988). *Fourth Report of the Independent Scientific Committee on Smoking and Health.* HMSO, London.

Jacob, J., Wilson, M., and Benowitz, N. L. (1981). Improved gas chromatographic method for the determination of nicotine and cotinine in biologic fluids. *Journal of Chromatography,* **222,** 61–70.

Saxen, I. (1974). Cleft lip and palate in Finland: parental histories, course of pregnancy and selected environmental factors. *International Journal of Epidemiology,* **3,** 263–70.

# 5. The effects of maternal cigarette smoking on placental structure and function in mid- to late gestation

*Graham J Burton*

Although the harmful effects of maternal cigarette smoking on the developing fetus have been extensively researched, surprisingly little attention has been paid to the placenta. The studies that have been performed generally fall into three categories:

1. Those describing the weight and macroscopic appearances of the organ at the time of delivery.
2. Those describing changes in its histological structure.
3. Those describing alterations in the organ's enzymatic and synthetic activities.

The findings in each of these three areas will be considered in turn, before discussing possible causative mechanisms.

## Placental weight and macroscopic appearances

Since the earliest reports that mean birth weight is reduced amongst women who smoke, many researchers have taken placental weight as a simple index of both the organ's well-being and its functional capacity. There is general agreement amongst those studies that have included sufficient cases to yield reliable data, that this index is unaffected by cigarette smoking (Mulcahy *et al*. 1970; Wilson 1971; Spira *et al*. 1975; Wingerd *et al*. 1976; Spira *et al*. 1977; Christianson 1979; Van der Veen and Fox 1982; Van der Velde and Treffers 1985). Consequently, there is an increase in the ratio between placental weight and birth weight—the so-called placental coefficient—amongst smokers.

When discussing the significance of these results, many authors inferred from the increase in the placental ratio that the organ undergoes some form of compensatory hypertrophy, and suggested that this is in response to chronic uterine hypoxia resulting from cigarette smoking. One might ask, however, why the degree of hypertrophy exhibited is insufficient to alleviate the reduction in birth weight, yet brings the placental weight into the middle of the range for normal pregnancies? A simpler, and perhaps more valid, conclusion might be that the placenta escapes the action of whatever factor it is that causes the decrease in birth weight amongst smokers. At present too little is known about the regulation of placental growth to justify further comment on this point.

Placental weight is a very poor indicator of placental well-being, however, because the volumes of maternal and fetal blood remaining in the organ after delivery are highly variable (Yao and Lind 1974; Bouw *et al.* 1976). It also gives no indication of the functional capabilities of the organ, as was illustrated by the recent stereological study of Jackson *et al.* (1987) on the influence of altitude on placental structure. Although no difference in mean placental weight was found between populations living at sea-level and 3600 m, considerable differences in the volumetric composition of the placentae from the two sample groups were observed. Notably, there was a significant reduction in the surface area of the villous tree at high altitude. Such internal changes could dramatically alter both the exchange and synthetic capabilities of the organ, and yet would go undetected by an analysis of placental weight alone.

On gross examination at delivery, smokers' placentae and membranes appear normal, with no alteration in the pattern of lobation or the incidence of maternal infarction (Mulcahy *et al.* 1970; Spira *et al.* 1977; Nordenvall *et al.* 1988). Indeed, it has been suggested that the frequency of such infarcts is lower amongst smokers than non-smokers (Christianson 1979).

There is, however, some dispute over the incidence of calcification observed in the region of the basal plate. Spira *et al.* (1977) found no difference in the occurrence of this lesion, whereas in the larger study of Christianson (1979), which included much heavier smokers, a higher incidence was observed amongst the smokers than the controls. Calcification is usually taken to be a sign of maturity or hypermaturity of the placenta, yet Christianson found the mean gestational age of the smokers' placentae to be slightly less than that of the non-smokers. It is therefore interesting that premature placental maturation and calcification has recently been diagnosed amongst both light and heavy smokers by ultrasonic techniques (Brown *et al.* 1988; Pinette *et al.* 1989). The clinical significance of this finding remains to be established, however, as no correlation was observed between the extent of these placental changes and the occurrence of small-for-gestational-age babies in the study of Brown *et al.* (1988).

## Histological appearances

At present it is uncertain how closely ultrasonic images of the placenta correlate with its histological structure. Confirming premature placental maturation histologically is made additionally difficult by the fact that all studies to date have been performed on placentae delivered at term. Thus, whilst Van der Veen and Fox (1982) found the villi to be of normal maturity in both smokers and non-smokers alike, examination of the placentae at, for example, 32 or 36 weeks gestation may yield different results.

Examination of the placenta at the light microscope level has generally not revealed a consistent pattern of changes attributable to maternal cigarette smoking. Undoubtedly, to a certain extent this reflects the heterogeneous nature of the organ, for it is now well recognized that marked regional variations in structure exist (Fox 1964; Teasdale 1978; Boyd *et al*. 1980; Bacon *et al*. 1986). Adequate sampling of a reasonable number of cases is thus required to obtain representative data, and suitable strategies were outlined by Mayhew and Burton (1988). In addition, few of the studies performed have applied quantitative techniques, and so the results have been largely descriptive. Consequently, within the literature there are numerous claims and counterclaims, and it is almost impossible to draw meaningful comparisons between the various published reports. Consideration will therefore be restricted to major findings, and in particular to those that may have significant physiological implications.

The general architecture of the villous tree within the smoker's placenta has been reported as normal, with no excess of villous inflammation or necrosis (Spira *et al*. 1977; Van der Veen and Fox 1982). Kaltenbach (1980) observed an increase in the total villous surface area, which was proportional to the number of cigarettes smoked (12.8 m² in non-smokers rising to 18.9 m² in those smoking 15–20 cigarettes per day). This was associated with an increase in the organ's weight from 558 g to 700 g ($n = 11$). The finding was not confirmed, however, by the study of the Van der Velde *et al*. (1983), whose proposed index of degree of villous branching actually relates directly to surface area, or by that of Teasdale and Ghislaine (1989). Indeed the results of the latter study indicated the reverse situation, with a reduced villous surface area amongst smokers, but the differences failed to attain statistical significance ($n = 5$).

In terms of villous structure the syncytiotrophoblast represents the outer covering of the villi, and is in contact with the maternal blood. It plays a key role in the active transport of nutrients between mother and fetus, and in the synthesis of many steroid and peptide hormones. For the most part it appears morphologically unaffected by maternal cigarette smoking, although small localized areas of microvillous damage and loss have been noted (Asmussen 1977; Van der Veen and Fox 1982). The disposition of the major syncytial organelles, such as mitochondria and endoplasmic reticulum, is similar to that in controls, but a reduction in the number of pinocytic vesicles and electron-dense secretory droplets has been reported in smokers' placentae (Asmussen 1980; Van der Veen and Fox 1982).

In the past much attention has been paid to the aggregation of syncytial nuclei into clumps known as syncytial knots. Some authors felt these were excessive in smokers' placentae (Spira *et al*. 1977; Kaltenbach 1980), whereas others did not (Naeye 1978; Van der Veen and Fox 1982; Van der Velde *et al*.

1983). The significance of syncytial knots in this context dates back to the *in vitro* work of Tominaga and Page (1966), who claimed that during organ culture of villi under hypoxic conditions a redistribution of the syncytium over the villous surface is achieved. This results in a thinning of the villous membrane over the capillaries, interpreted by the authors as facilitating gaseous exchange, and aggregation of the nuclei into knots over other parts of the villous surface. Subsequently, the finding of excessive syncytial knots in the smokers' placentae has been taken to support the idea that the organ is exposed to chronic hypoxia *in utero*. However, more recent work has shown that many instances of what appear histologically to be syncytial knots may be simple sectioning artifacts (Cantle *et al.* 1987), whilst more rigorous stereological studies have cast serious doubt on Tominaga and Page's interpretation of their data (Burton *et al.* 1989a; Ong and Burton 1991). These features can no longer be considered as evidence of adaptive changes, therefore.

Beneath the syncytiotrophoblast lie the cytotrophoblast cells, which represent a stem cell population capable of fusing with, and so regenerating, the syncytium (Boyd and Hamilton 1970). Proliferation of these cells, suggesting some form of accelerated repair, has been noted in the placentae of heavy smokers (Naeye 1978; Van der Veen and Fox 1982; Rush *et al.* 1986), but contradictory findings have also been presented (Asmussen 1977; Spira *et al.* 1977; Teasdale and Ghislaine 1989). The cytotrophoblast cells rest upon a well developed basal lamina and there appears to be general agreement that this displays an irregular thickening in the placentae of smokers (Asmussen 1977, 1980; Van der Veen and Fox 1982; Van der Velde *et al.* 1983, 1985). The significance of this change in terms of altered placental function however remains unclear.

This basal lamina represents the boundary between the trophoblast and the stromal core of the villus, and a prominent feature of the latter is the fetal capillary network. Because of its obvious key role in placental exchange considerable attention has been focused on the effects of maternal cigarette smoking upon this network. Reports again vary in the severity of the changes observed. Thus, both Asmussen (1977, 1980) and Mochizuki *et al.* (1984) noted a reduction in the degree of vascularity of the villi amongst heavy smokers, and suggested that this was due to a retardation in the growth of the capillary plexus. The capillaries that were present frequently displayed irregular luminal margins, and apical blebs arising from the endothelial cells were a conspicuous feature in these studies. Other studies have confirmed that the calibre of the capillary network is reduced in smokers' placentae, but have not supported the idea that the actual number of vessels present is decreased (Van der Veen and Fox 1982; Copius Peereboom-Stegeman *et al.* 1983). At the other end of the spectrum are those reports that have concluded there are no effects of cigarette smoking upon the fetal vasculature (Spira *et al.* 1977; Kaltenbach 1980; Teasdale and Ghislaine 1989).

One of the main problems when assessing the postpartum placenta, however, is that the fetal capillary network is inevitably partially collapsed, to a variable and unpredictable degree. This is a consequence of both the placental transfusion, a major shift of extracorporeal blood back to the fetus at the time of delivery, and leakage of fetal blood from sites of damage caused to the villous tree by the rigours of the delivery. The luminal margins of the capillaries are therefore bound to appear irregular, and this effect is likely to be more pronounced if vasoactive compounds such as nicotine are present. In an attempt to overcome this problem perfusion–fixation has been applied to the placenta, for by using physiological pressures it is possible to redistend the capillaries to their *in vivo* dimensions (Burton *et al*. 1987; Feneley and Burton 1991). When this technique was applied to smokers' placentae the endothelial cell profiles appeared normal and only a small, yet statistically significant, reduction in the proportion of the villi occupied by the fetal capillaries was observed (33.6 per cent in heavy smokers (> 15 cigarettes per day) compared to 37.6 per cent in controls) (Burton *et al*. 1989*b*). This was much less than the almost 50 per cent reduction reported by Van der Velde *et al*. (1983), and more in line with the findings of normality by Kaltenbach (1980) and Teasdale and Ghislaine (1989). However, it must be remembered that even a modest reduction in blood vessel calibre can have profound physiological consequences, as the rate of flow through a vessel is proportional to the fourth power of its radius. Interestingly, Doppler studies performed *in utero* have shown that the fetal placental vasculature may show transient periods (15 min duration) of vasoconstriction after the smoking of just one cigarette by the mother (Morrow *et al*. 1988).

Intimately associated with the fetal capillaries are the vasculosyncytial membranes, which are points where locally dilated vessels come into close contact with the overlying trophoblast. As the villous membrane is particularly thin at these sites, they are generally thought to be the principal areas for gaseous exchange across the placenta (Fox 1967; Ludwig 1972). It is thus of considerable interest that both Van der Veen and Fox (1982) and Copius Peereboom-Stegeman *et al*. (1983) noted a reduction in the frequency of these specializations in the placentae of smokers. The appearance of vasculosyncytial membranes in sectioned material is known, however, to be heavily influenced by the degree of distension of the underlying fetal capillary network, and so indirectly by the fixation techniques employed (Bouw *et al*. 1976; Voigt *et al*. 1978; Burton *et al*. 1987; Feneley and Burton 1991).

It is also now realized that the number of vasculosyncytial membranes present alone is not a very informative index of the placenta's functional capacity for diffusional exchange, as it takes no account of their areal extent (Mayhew and Burton 1988). Much more relevant is the mean thickness of the villous membrane, and in particular the harmonic mean thickness, for being based on the reciprocals of the local thicknesses this emphasizes the presence of the vasculosyncytial membranes (Laga *et al*. 1973; Mayhew *et al*. 1984, 1986). As yet the only study to provide such estimates for the smokers' placentae is that of Burton *et al.* (1989*b*), who reported a statistically significant increase in the harmonic mean thickness from 3.6 μm in the controls to 4.2 μm in the placentae of mothers who smoked more than 15 cigarettes per day. On the morphometric model of Mayhew *et al.* (1986) this change would be responsible for an approximate 10 per cent reduction in the organ's diffusing capacity.

Whether this reduction is in any way causal of the diminution in birth weight seen amongst smokers is difficult to determine, as changes in other systems, for example an increase in the fetal haematocrit or rate of blood flow (Alverson *et al.* 1986), may be sufficient to compensate and so maintain fetal supply. The decreased diffusion capacity may, however, compound other adverse changes induced by cigarette smoking, such as a diminished uteroplacental circulation, and so it is difficult to predict accurately the consequences *in vivo*. Interestingly, identical changes were observed in the placentae of women who gave up smoking early in gestation. A strong test to determine the clinical significance of these changes would therefore be to examine birthweight in this population. At present there seems little evidence to suggest that cessation of smoking in early pregnancy has any positive impact on birthweight (for a discussion see Chapter 15).

When reviewing these macroscopic and histological findings it is clear that, with the exception of the vascular changes, the majority of smokers' placentae appear remarkably normal. However, despite this apparent normality, evidence is emerging of significant damage at the genetic level, for maternal smoking is associated with the bonding of three specific adducts (chemical addition products) to placental DNA (Everson *et al.* 1988). As yet it is not clear whether this placental binding plays any role in the impairment of fetal development, or whether it merely parallels other more significant biochemical changes, either in the placenta or the fetus. Previous work in mice has confirmed a close association between the finding of DNA adducts in the placenta and their presence in many fetal organs, such as the heart, liver, and brain (Randerath *et al.* 1986).

## Enzymatic and synthetic changes

Biochemical investigations have revealed disturbances in placental function associated with cigarette smoking, perhaps the most important of which is a reduction in the active uptake of amino acids from the maternal blood. Consequently, the concentrations of several essential and non-essential amino acids are lower in the placental villi of women who smoke compared to non-smoking controls (Sastry *et al.* 1987).

Other receptor-mediated mechanisms have also been shown to be influenced by cigarette smoking. For example, it has been demonstrated that the activity of epidermal growth factor (EGF)-stimulated kinase activity is markedly depressed in smokers, owing to the absence of a specific receptor protein (Wang *et al.* 1988). The significance of this finding remains uncertain, as the role of EGF in placental development and differentiation has yet to be fully elucidated.

The synthetic activities of the syncytiotrophoblast are influenced in different ways depending on the hormone in question. Levels of human chorionic gonadotrophin in the maternal serum are reduced amongst smokers during the second trimester (Bernstein *et al.* 1989; Cuckle *et al.* 1990). By contrast, during the third trimester maternal levels of human placental lactogen are within the normal range or even slightly elevated (Moser *et al.* 1974; Spellacy *et al.* 1976), although recent evidence suggests any increase is dependent upon the sex of the fetus (Bremme *et al.* 1990). As levels of this hormone are considered to be the most efficient biochemical test of placental function currently available (Westergaard *et al.* 1986), these findings argue against major disruption of the syncytiotrophoblast as a consequence of maternal cigarette smoking.

Not surprisingly, induction of enzyme systems capable of oxidizing polycyclic aromatic hydrocarbons has been shown to result from both direct and passive smoking, and these again have been localized to the syncytiotrophoblast (e.g. Pasanen *et al.* 1988; Huel *et al.* 1989).

## Possible causative factors

In the past many authors have linked the changes they observed to a state of chronic uterine hypoxia, resulting from either a reduction in the uterine blood flow or the effects of elevated maternal levels of carboxyhaemoglobin. This idea was supported by the finding that nicotine administered to pregnant Rhesus monkeys causes a severe reduction in uterine artery blood flow (Suzuki *et al.* 1980). Doppler studies performed on women have confirmed that cigarette smoking causes not only a marked transient decrease in uteroplacental blood flow, but also a more subtle chronic reduction (Lehtovirta and Forss 1978; Andersen and Hermann 1984).

Whilst a degree of uterine ischaemia could account for some of the morphological changes observed in smokers' placentae, such as cytotrophoblastic hyperplasia, trophoblastic basal lamina thickening, and decreased syncytial pinocytic activity, not all the findings can be explained on this basis (Fox and Jones 1983). Subsequent to their review it has also become apparent that the placenta is capable of adapting to low oxygen tensions by a thinning of the villous membrane at certain sites, leading to a reduction in the harmonic mean thickness (Critchley and Burton 1987; Jackson *et al.* 1988). The finding of an increased membrane thickness amongst smokers' placentae is thus contrary to expectations based on this model.

Other factors, therefore, must be responsible for certain of the changes, and particular attention has been paid to cadmium, as high levels have been detected in the placentae of smoking mothers (Miller and Gardner 1981; Van Hattum *et al.* 1981; Kuhnert *et al.* 1987a). When cadmium chloride is injected subcutaneously into pregnant rats a high incidence of fetal death results (75 per cent), yet fetal tissue levels are only minimally elevated. Conversely, when the fetuses are injected directly *in utero*, then the fetal death rate remains relatively low (11.5 per cent) despite tissue levels far in excess of those associated with the fetal deaths following maternal injection (Levin and Miller 1980).

These surprising findings demonstrate that the fetotoxic effects of cadmium must be exerted either through changes in the placenta or through changes in the mother. The injection studies also revealed that the chorio-allantoic placenta of the rat accumulates cadmium very avidly, and to a higher level than other organs (Levin *et al.* 1981).

Daily administration of cadmium to pregnant rats has a profound effect upon the placental vasculature, resulting in a reduction in the fractional volume of the fetal vessels and an increase in the villous membrane thickness (Copius Peereboom-Stegeman *et al.* 1983). These changes are qualitatively very similar to those observed in smokers' placentae.

Cadmium may also have an influence on the transport activities of the placenta, as it acts as an antagonist to zinc in zinc-requiring metaloenzymes, such as alkaline phosphatase. In addition, it appears that the binding of cadmium to placental tissues can also lead to a sequestration of zinc, with the result that levels of zinc in the fetal erythrocytes are lower in mothers who smoke than in controls (Kuhnert *et al.* 1987*b*). Consequently, the activity of metaloenzymes in the fetus may also be depressed.

Cigarette smoke, however, contains many hundreds of potential toxins, to which the developing placenta is exposed. Many of these have not been fully characterized, and their influences on placental structure and function have certainly not been assessed. It is therefore impossible to determine the precise cause of the placental changes observed in smokers, but it seems most likely that they result from a combination of uterine ischaemia and toxic damage. Fortunately, it is apparent from the study of Burton *et al.* (1989*b*) that if women stop smoking before conceiving their placentae are macroscopically and microscopically normal. Any potentially placentotoxic agent must therefore be cleared fairly rapidly from the maternal bloodstream. Conversely, if mothers stop smoking during the first trimester then the placentae are identical in terms of the changes in the fetal vasculature and membrane thickness to those of continuing smokers. These findings further support the argument that nicotine-induced uterine ischaemia is not the sole causative factor, for nicotine is not accumulated by the placenta (Suzuki *et al.* 1974) and so levels may be expected to return to normal soon after cessation of smoking. Cadmium levels may be slower to fall, but further studies are required to confirm this point.

It is notable that many studies have failed to demonstrate a dose–response relationship between the number of cigarettes smoked and the changes observed. This most probably reflects the inaccuracies of mothers' accounts of their smoking habits. Correlations with biochemical assays of cigarette exposure may be more fruitful, as was the case in the study of Everson *et al.* (1988).

## Other aspects of placentation

So far, only changes in the placental disc have been considered, but there are other complications of pregnancy in which a disturbance in the normal interaction between trophoblast and endometrium may prove to play a significant role. For example, the incidence of both placenta previa and abruptio placentae is raised amongst smokers (Meyer and Tonascia 1977), and a strong positive correlation exists between the duration of maternal smoking prior to the pregnancy and the occurrence of one or other of these complications (Naeye 1979). As the bases of these conditions are at present unknown it is impossible to speculate how they may be influenced by maternal cigarette smoking. A much more detailed understanding of the normal process of implantation is necessary before these questions can be addressed.

## Conclusion

From this review of published findings it is obvious that no clear pattern of changes is seen in the placentae of women who smoke during pregnancy. Morphologically, it seems that the placenta is neither growth-retarded nor hypertrophied, that the surface area and general architecture of the villous tree is normal and that, with the possible exceptions of a slightly excessive incidence of focal syncytial necrosis and a decrease in pinocytic activity, the trophoblast appears healthy. There is general agreement that the trophoblastic basement membrane shows irregular thickening, and that the fetal capillaries have a reduced calibre, which may result in a decrease in the diffusional capacity of the organ.

Overall, however, it might be justifiably concluded that the placenta appears remarkably normal, and any localized damage of the trophoblast would seem to be well within the repair capabilities of the organ. It is clear, therefore, that the reduction in birth weight of the babies of smokers can not be attributed to any gross disruption of placental development or differentiation. Biochemically, there is some evidence of interference with transport mechanisms, and this, along with a deficient oxygen and nutrient supply to the uterus, may play a more major role.

## References

Alverson, D. C., Eldridge, M., Dillon, T., Blomquist, T., and Berman, W. (1986). Pulsed Doppler evaluation of the fetal and neonatal circulation. In *Fetal physiological measurements*, (ed. P. Rolfe), pp. 236–47. Butterworths, London.

Andersen, K. V. and Hermann, N. (1984). Placenta flow reduction in pregnant smokers. *Acta Obstetrica et Gynecologica Scandinavica*, **63**, 707–9.

Asmussen, I. (1977). Ultrastructure of the human placenta at term. Observations on placentas from newborn children of smoking and non-smoking mothers. *Acta Obstetrica et Gynecologica Scandinavica*, **56**, 119–26.

Asmussen, I. (1980). Ultrastructure of the villi and fetal capillaries in placentas from smoking and non-smoking mothers. *British Journal of Obstetrics and Gynaecology*, **87**, 239–45.

Bacon, B. J., Gilbert, R. D., and Longo, L. D. (1986). Regional anatomy of the term human placenta. *Placenta*, **7**, 233–41.

Bernstein, L., Pike, M. C., Lobo, R. A., Depue, R. H., Ross, R. K., and Henderson, B. E. (1989). Cigarette smoking in pregnancy results in marked decrease in maternal hCG and oestradiol levels. *British Journal of Obstetrics and Gynaecology*, **96**, 92–6.

Bouw, G. M., Stolte, L. A. M., Baak, J. P. A., and Oort, J. (1976). Quantitative morphology of the placenta. 1. Standardization of sampling. *European Journal of Obstetrics and Gynecology and Reproductive Biology*, **6**, 325–31.

Boyd, J. D. and Hamilton, W. J. (1970). *The human placenta*. Heffer, Cambridge.

Boyd, P. A., Brown, R. A., and Stewart, W. J. (1980). Quantitative structural differences within the normal term human placenta: A pilot study. *Placenta*, **1**, 337–44.

Bremme, K., Lagerström, M., Andersson, O., Johansson, S., and Eneroth, P. (1990). Influences of maternal smoking and fetal sex on maternal serum oestriol, prolactin, hCG, and hPL levels. *Archives of Gynecology and Obstetrics*, **247**, 95–103.

Brown, H. L., Miller, J. M., Khawli, D., and Gabert, H. A. (1988). Premature placental calcification in maternal cigarette smokers. *Obstetrics and Gynecology*, **71**, 914–17.

Burton, G. J., Ingram, S. C., and Palmer, M. E. (1987). The influence of mode of fixation on morphometrical data derived from terminal villi in the human placenta at term: A comparison of immersion and perfusion fixation. *Placenta*, **8**, 37–51.

Burton, G. J., Mayhew, T. M., and Robertson, L. A. (1989*a*). Stereological re-examination of the effects of varying oxygen tensions on human placental villi maintained in organ culture for up to 12 h. *Placenta*, **10**, 263–73.

Burton, G. J., Palmer, M. E., and Dalton, K. J. (1989*b*). Morphometric differences between the placental vasculature of non-smokers, smokers and ex-smokers. *British Journal of Obstetrics and Gynaecology*, **96**, 907–15.

Cantle, S. J., Kaufmann, P., Luckhardt, M., and Schweikhart, G. (1987). Interpretation of syncytial sprouts and bridges in the human placenta. *Placenta*, **8**, 221–34.

Christianson, R. E. (1979). Gross differences observed in the placentas of smokers and nonsmokers. *American Journal of Epidemiology*, **110**, 178–87.

Copius Peereboom-Stegeman, J. H. J., Van der Velde, W. J., and Dessing, J. W. M. (1983). Influence of cadmium on placental structure. *Ecotoxicology and Environmental Safety*, **7**, 79–86.

Critchley, G. R. and Burton, G. J. (1987). Intra-lobular variations in barrier thickness in the mature human placenta. *Placenta*, **8**, 185–94.

Cuckle, H. S., Wald, N. J., Densem, J. W., Royston, P., Knight, G. J., Haddow, J. E., and Canick, J. A. (1990). The effect of smoking in pregnancy on maternal serum alpha-fetoprotein, unconjugated oestriol, human chorionic gonadotrophin, progesterone and dehydroepiandrosterone sulphate levels. *British Journal of Obstetrics and Gynaecology*, **97**, 272–6.

Everson, R. B., Randerath, E., Santella, R. M., Avitts, T. A., Weinstein, I. B., and

Randerath, K. (1988). Quantitative associations between DNA damage in human placenta and maternal smoking and birth weight. *Journal National Cancer Institute,* **80,** 567–76.

Feneley, M. R. and Burton, G. J. (1991). Villous composition and membrane thickness in the human placenta at term: A stereological study using unbiased estimators and optimal fixation techniques. *Placenta,* **12,** 131–42.

Fox, H. (1964). The pattern of villous variability in the normal placenta. *Journal of Obstetrics and Gynaecology of the British Commonwealth,* **71,** 749–58.

Fox, H. (1967). The incidence and significance of vasculosyncytial membranes in the human placenta. *Journal of Obstetrics and Gynaecology of the British Commonwealth,* **74,** 28–33.

Fox, H. and Jones, C. J. P. (1983). Pathology of trophoblast. In *Biology of trophoblast,* (ed. Y. W. Loke and A. Whyte), pp. 137–85. Elsevier, Amsterdam.

Huel, G., Godin, J., Moreau, T., Girard, F., Sahuquillo, J., Hellier, G., *et al.* (1989). Aryl hydrocarbon hydroxylase activity in human placenta of passive smokers. *Environmental Research,* **50,** 173–83.

Jackson, M. R., Mayhew, T. M., and Haas, J. D. (1987). The volumetric composition of human term placentae: Altitudinal, ethnic and sex differences in Bolivia. *Journal of Anatomy,* **152,** 173–87.

Jackson, M. R., Mayhew, T. M., and Haas, J. D. (1988). On the factors which contribute to thinning of the villous membrane in human placentae at high altitude. I. Thinning and regional variation in thickness of trophoblast. *Placenta,* **9,** 1–8.

Kaltenbach, F. J. (1980). The relation of placental morphology to hormonal status in pre-eclampsia and in women who smoke. *Proceedings of the Serono Symposia,* **35,** 329–37.

Kuhnert, B. R., Kuhnert, P. M., Debanne, S., and Williams, T. G. (1987*a*). The relationship between cadmium, zinc, and birth weight in pregnant women who smoke. *American Journal of Obstetrics and Gynecology,* **157,** 1247–51.

Kuhnert, P. M., Kuhnert, B. R., Erhard, B. S., Brashear, W. T., Groh-Wargo, S. L., and Webster, S. (1987*b*). The effect of smoking on placental and fetal zinc status. *American Journal of Obstetrics and Gynecology,* **157,** 1241–6.

Laga, E. M., Driscoll, S. G., and Munro, H. N. (1973). Quantitative studies of human placenta. I. Morphometry. *Biology of the Neonate,* **23,** 231–59.

Lehtovirta, P. and Forss, M. (1978). The acute effect of smoking on intervillous blood flow of the placenta. *British Journal of Obstetrics and Gynaecology,* **85,** 729–31.

Levin, A. A. and Miller, R. K. (1980). Fetal toxicity of cadmium in the rat: maternal vs fetal injections. *Teratology,* **22,** 1–5.

Levin, A. A., Plautz, J. R., and Di Sant'Agnese, P. A. (1981). Cadmium: placental mechanisms of fetal toxicity. *Placenta,* (**Suppl. 3**), 303–18.

Ludwig, K. S. (1972). The morphologic structure of the placenta in relation to its exchange function. In *Respiratory gas exchange and blood flow in the placenta,* (ed. L. D. Longo and H. Bartels), pp. 13–21. US Department of Health, Education and Welfare, Bethesda, Maryland.

Mayhew, T. M. and Burton, G. J. (1988). Methodological problems in placental morphometry: Apologia for the use of stereology based on sound sampling practice. *Placenta,* **9,** 565–81.

Mayhew, T. M., Joy, C. F., and Haas, J. D. (1984). Structure-function correlation in the human placenta: The morphometric diffusing capacity for oxygen at full term. *Journal of Anatomy,* **139,** 691–708.

Mayhew, T. M., Jackson, M. R., and Haas, J. D. (1986). Microscopical morphology of the human placenta and its effects on oxygen diffusion: A morphometric model. *Placenta*, **7**, 121–31.

Meyer, M. B. and Tonascia, J. A. (1977). Maternal smoking, pregnancy complications, and perinatal mortality. *American Journal of Obstetrics and Gynecology*, **128**, 494–502.

Miller, R. K. and Gardner, K. A. (1981). Cadmium in the human placenta: Relationship to smoking. *Teratology*, **23**, 51A.

Mochizuki, M., Maruo, T., Masuko, K., and Ohtsu, T. (1984). Effects of smoking on fetoplacental-maternal system during pregnancy. *American Journal of Obstetrics and Gynecology*, **149**, 413–20.

Morrow, R. J., Knox Ritchie, J. W., and Bull, S. B. (1988). Maternal cigarette smoking: The effects on umbilical and uterine blood flow velocity. *American Journal of Obstetrics and Gynecology*, **159**, 1069–71.

Moser, R. J., Hollingsworth, D. R., Carlson, J. W., and Lamotte, L. (1974). Human chorionic somatomammotropin in normal adolescent primiparous pregnancy. 1. Effect of smoking. *American Journal of Obstetrics and Gynecology*, **120**, 1080–6.

Mulcahy, R., Murphy, J., and Martin, F. (1970). Placental changes and maternal weight in smoking and nonsmoking mothers. *American Journal of Obstetrics and Gynecology*, **106**, 703–4.

Naeye, R. L. (1978). Effects of maternal cigarette smoking on the fetus and placenta. *British Journal of Obstetrics and Gynaecology*, **85**, 732–7.

Naeye, R. L. (1979). The duration of maternal cigarette smoking, fetal and placental disorders. *Early Human Development*, **3**, 229–37.

Nordenvall, M., Sandstedt, B., and Ulmsten, U. (1988). Relationship between placental shape, cord insertion, lobes and gestational outcome. *Acta Obstetrica et Gynecologica Scandinavica*, **67**, 611–16.

Ong, P. J. L. and Burton, G. J. (1991). Thinning of the placental villous membrane during hypoxic organ culture: Structural adaptation or syncytial degeneration? *European Journal of Obstetrics and Gynecology and Reproductive Biology*, **39**, 103–10.

Pasanen, M., Stenback, F., Park, S. S., Gelboin, H. V., and Pelkonen, O. (1988). Immunohistochemical detection of human placental cytochrome P-450 associated mono-oxygenase system inducible by maternal cigarette smoking. *Placenta*, **9**, 267–75.

Pinette, M. G., Loftus-Brault, K., Nardi, D. A., and Rodis, J. F. (1989). Maternal smoking and accelerated placental maturation. *Obstetrics and Gynecology*, **73**, 379–82.

Randerath, E., Avitts, T. A., Reddy, M. V., Miller, R. H., Everson, R. B., and Randerath, K. (1986). Comparative [32]P-analysis of cigarette smoke-induced DNA damage in human tissues and mouse skin. *Cancer Research*, **46**, 5869–77.

Rush, D., Kristal, A., Blanc, W., Navarro, C., Chauhan, P., Campbell Brown, M. *et al.* (1986). The effects of maternal cigarette smoking on placental morphology, histomorphometry, and biochemistry. *American Journal of Perinatology*, **3**, 263–72.

Sastry, B. V. R., Janson, V. E., Boehm, F. H., Ahmed, M., Knots, J., and Schinfeld, J. S. (1987). Maternal smoking depresses amino acid uptake by human placenta. *Federation Proceedings*, **46**, 3750.

Spellacy, W. N., Buhi, W. C., and Birk, S. A. (1976). The effect of smoking on serum placental lactogen levels. *American Journal of Obstetrics and Gynecology*, **127**, 232–4.

Spira, A., Spira, N., Goujard, J., and Schwartz, D. (1975). Smoking during pregnancy and placental weight. A multivariate analysis on 3759 cases. *Journal of Perinatal Medicine*, **3**, 237–41.

Spira, A., Philippe, E., Spira, N., Dreyfus, J., and Schwartz, D. (1977). Smoking during pregnancy and placental pathology. *Biomedicine*, **27**, 266–70.

Suzuki, K., Horigushi, T., Comas-Urrutia, A. C., Mueller-Heubach, E., Morishima, H. O., and Adamsons, K. (1974). Placental transfer and distribution of nicotine in the pregnant rhesus monkey. *American Journal of Obstetrics and Gynecology*, **119**, 253–62.

Suzuki, K., Minei, L. J., and Johnson, E. E. (1980). Effect of nicotine upon uterine blood flow in the pregnant rhesus monkey. *American Journal of Obstetrics and Gynecology*, **136**, 1009–13.

Teasdale, F. (1978). Functional significance of the zonal morphologic differences in the normal human placenta. A morphometric study. *American Journal of Obstetrics and Gynecology*, **130**, 773–81.

Teasdale, F. and Ghislaine, J-J. (1989). Morphological changes in the placentas of smoking mothers: A histomorphometric study. *Biology of the Neonate*, **55**, 251–9.

Tominaga, T. and Page, E. W. (1966). Accommodation of the human placenta to hypoxia. *American Journal of Obstetrics and Gynecology*, **94**, 679–91.

Van der Veen, F. and Fox, H. (1982). The effects of cigarette smoking on the human placenta: A light and electron microscopic study. *Placenta*, **3**, 243–56.

Van der Velde, W. J., Copius Peereboom-Stegeman, J. H. J., Treffers, P. E., and James, J. (1983). Structural changes in the placenta of smoking mothers: A quantitative study. *Placenta*, **4**, 231–40.

Van der Velde, W. J. and Treffers, P. E. (1985). Smoking in pregnancy: The influence on percentile birth weight, mean birth weight, placental weight, menstrual age, perinatal mortality and maternal diastolic blood pressure. *Gynecologic and Obstetric Investigation*, **19**, 57–63.

Van der Velde, W. J., Copius Peereboom-Stegeman, J. H. J., Treffers, P. E., and James, J. (1985). Basal lamina thickening in the placentae of smoking mothers. *Placenta*, **6**, 329–40.

Van Hattum, B., de Voogt, P., and Copius Peereboom, J. W. (1981). An analytical procedure for the determination of cadmium in human placentae. *International Journal of Environmental Analytical Chemistry*, **10**, 121–33.

Voigt, S., Kaufmann, P., and Schweikhart, G. (1978). Zur abgrenzung normaler, artefizieller und pathologischer strukturen in reifen menschlichen plazentazotten. I. Morphometrische Untersuchungen Zum Einflub Des Fixationsmodus. *Archiv fur Gynakologie*, **226**, 347–62.

Wang, S. L., Lucier, G. W., Everson, R. B., Sunahara, G. I., and Shiverick, K. T. (1988). Smoking-related alterations in epidermal growth factor and insulin receptors in human placenta. *Molecular Pharmacology*, **34**, 265–71.

Westergaard, J. G., Teisner, B., and Grudzinskas, J. G. (1986). Biochemical assessment of placental function—late pregnancy. *Clinics in Obstetrics and Gynaecology*, **13**, No. 3, 571–91.

Wilson, E. W. (1971). The effect of smoking in pregnancy on the placental coefficient. *New Zealand Medical Journal*, **74**, 384–5.

Wingerd, J., Christianson, R., Lovitt, W. V., and Schoen, E. J. (1976). Placental ratio in white and black women: Relation to smoking and anemia. *American Journal of Obstetrics and Gynecology*, **124**, 671–5.

Yao, A. C. and Lind, J. (1974). Blood flow in the umbilical vessels during the third stage of labour. *Biology of the Neonate*, **25**, 186–93.

# 6. The effect of smoking on oxygen transfer and placental circulation

*E Malcolm Symonds*

The important structural component of the placenta is the chorionic villus, for it is at this level that the fetus has its most intimate contact with the maternal circulation; it is here that nutrient transfer and gaseous exchange occurs. The chorionic villi develop over the decidua basalis, initially from main stem villi, which subsequently split into a series of second- and third-order stems. These stems may also subdivide to form minor villous stems, which are called anchoring villi. This pattern of division and growth vastly increases the available space for gaseous transfer.

## Histological structure of the mature villus

By full term, the syncytial thickness has a mean value of 6.5 $\mu$ but may contain areas of considerable variation. There are also 'sprouts', 'buds', 'knots', and 'proliferation' nodes. At full term, cytotrophoblast has effectively disappeared. The villous cores contain the functional vascular elements vital to the function of the placenta. The mesenchyme is separated from the overlying trophoblast by the basement membrane. The stromal cells are fibroblasts and Hofbauer cells lie in the interstices. These cells are also probably of mesenchymal origin. Their function remains obscure but they may be involved in transport mechanisms (see also Chapter 5).

Maturation of the branch villi during the course of placental ageing is associated with thinning of the syncytiotrophoblast and the formation of organelle-poor alpha syncytium. This enhances the transfer of gases and nutrients, whereas the cells lining the stem villi remain thick and rich in organelles, are known as the beta syncytium, and are concerned predominantly with synthetic activities rather than transfer mechanisms. Examination of the ultrastructure of the human placental barrier (Fig. 6.1) (Begley *et al.* 1980) shows that in the mature placenta the only separation between the fetal and maternal circulations consists of the syncytiotrophoblast, the fetal endothelium and a thin layer of intervening connective tissue.

## Oxygen and carbon dioxide transport in normal pregnancy

Oxygen diffuses readily across the placental barrier but in passing through the

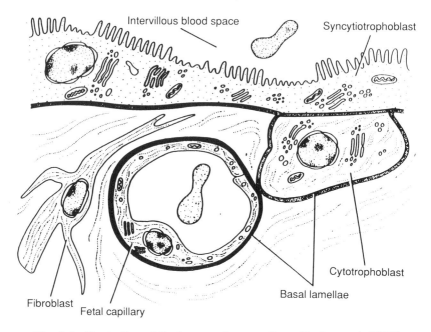

**Fig. 6.1.** Illustration of the human placenta. From Begley *et al*. (1980).

placenta some 20 per cent of the oxygen is extracted for metabolism of the syncytiotrophoblasts. The pressure gradient between the maternal and fetal circulations is, therefore, misleading if the Fick principle is applied and oxygen is about four times more diffusible than implied by venous partial pressure differences. The level of oxygen dissolved in plasma determines the diffusion gradient and the direction and rate of transfer, although the major oxygen content of fetal blood is linked to oxyhaemoglobin. Fetal blood with a high haemoglobin concentration has an increased oxygen carrying capacity and the transfer of oxygen to the fetus is further facilitated by the high affinity of fetal haemoglobin for oxygen. The oxygen dissociation curve for fetal haemoglobin is shifted to the left of the curve for adult haemoglobin and a small change in the partial pressure of oxygen causes a larger change in oxygen saturation in the fetal blood than would occur in maternal blood.

Further, the double Bohr effect results in changes that facilitate the transfer of oxygen to the fetus. A fall in maternal pH results in a reduced oxygen affinity whereas the transfer of carbon dioxide from the fetal to maternal circulation increases the pH of fetal blood and hence the affinity of fetal haemoglobin for oxygen.

## The transfer of carbon dioxide

The diffusion of carbon dioxide also depends on the diffusion gradient across the placental membrane and the fetal and maternal uteroplacental blood flow. However, carbon dioxide is far more soluble than oxygen. The difference in partial carbon dioxide pressure is less than for oxygen because diffusion is more rapid. Carbon dioxide is carried predominantly as bicarbonate, with 60 per cent carried in this form, 30 per cent as carbamino complexes, such as with haemoglobin and plasma proteins, and only 10 per cent in physical solution. Bicarbonate ions, as such, do not cross the placenta in any significant quantity. The oxygenation of fetal blood promotes the release of $H^+$ ions, which promotes the release of carbon dioxide. With this transfer, bicarbonate ions are lost in the fetus and found in the mother. Maternal erythrocyte carbonic anhydrase activity is significantly higher than in the fetus.

## The effect of smoking on oxygen transfer to the fetus

The adverse effects of smoking on the fetus derive principally from:

1. The inhalation of carbon monoxide and its interference with oxygen availability.
2. The effect of nicotine on the uteroplacental vasculature as a vasoconstrictor.

### The effect of carbon monoxide on the fetus

Carbon monoxide (CO) is found extensively in the external environment. It is colourless, odourless, and combines with high affinity to haemoglobin. It has an affinity 200 times greater than oxygen and therefore displaces oxygen from protohaem, which is a ferrous iron complex of protoporphyrin IX. The linkage to carbon monoxide is reversible. Longo (1977), in reviewing the effect of carbon monoxide in healthy individuals has shown that carboxy-haemoglobin levels as low as 4 to 5 per cent may result in significant effects on vital functions. Typical concentrations of carbon monoxide are shown in Fig. 6.2. These may range from as low as 0.06–0.5 parts per million in sea air to 30 000 to 80 000 in automobile exhaust and up to 60 000 parts per million in cigarette smoke. The alveolar concentration in smoke has been estimated at 300–400 parts per million. There is also some endogenous production of carbon monoxide generated from the protoporphyrin ring to form carbon monoxide and bilirubin, but these values are very low, with production rates of 0.42 ml of carbon monoxide (CO) per hour in men, similar values during the proliferative phase of the menstrual cycle in women, but values twice as high in the progestational phase and during pregnancy. The blood carboxy-haemoglobin concentration ([HbCO]) (saturation) is expressed as:

$$[HbCO] = \frac{\text{blood CO content}}{\text{blood CO capacity}} \times 100$$

Douglas *et al.* (1912) showed that the ratio between carboxyhaemoglobin and oxyhaemoglobin ($HbO_2$) is determined by the partial pressures of carbon

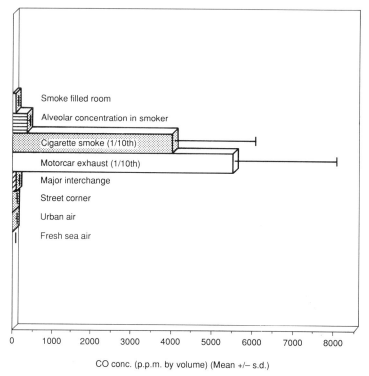

**Fig. 6.2.** Concentrations of carbon monoxide in various environs expressed in parts per million (data derived from Robinson and Robbins 1970).

monoxide and oxygen ($O_2$) and by an affinity factor (M). This relationship is expressed as follows:

$$\frac{[HbCO]}{[HbO_2]} = \frac{PCO \times M}{PO_2}$$

where $PCO$ is partial carbon monoxide pressure and $PO_2$ is partial oxygen pressure. M is an expression of the relative affinity of haemoglobin for carbon monoxide as compared with oxygen.

Roughton and Darling, in 1944, showed that carbon monoxide shifts the oxygen dissociation curve to the left in the both maternal and fetal blood.

*Time course changes and carbon monoxide transfer*    Longo and Hill (1977) measured fetal haemoglobin concentrations in fetal lambs in chronically cannulated animals in order to examine the rate of change in carboxyhaemoglobin saturation in the fetal lamb in response to maternal administration of 30–330 p.p.m. carbon monoxide. Maternal levels of carboxyhaemoglobin increased rapidly over the first 2–3 h and reached equilibrium after 7–8 h. The half-time to maximum concentration was 2.5 h. Fetal levels increased more slowly than maternal values with little change over the first hour, a slow increase for the next 4–5 h, but reaching equilibrium at 5–6 h. However, steady-state equilibrium was not reached for 36 to 48 h; the half-time was 7 h. It is likely that the washout time follows the opposite pattern, with fetal carbon monoxide elimination lagging behind maternal values, although clearly these data are not available in human subjects.

*The effect of maternal smoking*   The relationship between maternal and fetal carboxyhaemoglobin levels in women who smoke has been reported in several studies. In the eight studies reported on this subject and reviewed by Longo (1977), fetal (HbCO) saturation varied from 2.4 to 7.6 per cent and maternal level from 2.0 to 8.3 per cent, levels which are 6 to 7 times higher than those seen in non-pregnant females. The variation established in these reports can be explained by the different sampling times in relation to the time of delivery.

Numerous studies have now demonstrated that smoking during pregnancy reduces the birth weight of the infant and Miller and Hassanein (1974) have also shown that crown–heel length is reduced. The baby is, therefore, generally small. These findings are, of course, not necessarily a cause for concern for the individual baby unless there is an increase in perinatal mortality or subsequent developmental impairment. Allowing for additional factors, such as age, parity, race, and social status, it is now generally agreed that the perinatal death rate is increased as a direct effect of smoking. Meyer and Comstock (1972) quantified this increase in risk at 20 per cent for those women smoking up to 20 cigarettes per day and 35 per cent in women smoking in excess of one packet of cigarettes per day.

Smoking also diminishes fetal breathing *in utero*, and the studies of Gennser *et al.* (1975) demonstrated a reduction of 15 per cent in the time of respiratory movements. It is not certain what the mechanism of these changes is, and it cannot be directly attributed to changes in carboxyhaemoglobin levels.

The studies of Asmussen and Kjeldsen (1975) on the human umbilical artery showed significant changes in the vasculature in mothers who smoked during pregnancy and their studies revealed evidence of swollen and irregular endothelial cells with unusual 'cobblestone' appearances as well as cytoplasmic blebs or protrusions on the endothelial surface. Transmission electron microscopy studies also showed evidence of endothelial swelling, dilation of rough endoplasmic reticulum, extensive subendothelial oedema, and abnormal appearance of the lysosomes. There was also loss of collagen fibres. From his review of the literature, Longo (1977) concluded that fetal carboxyhaemoglobin concentrations are 10–15 per cent greater than in the mother and that carbon monoxide uptake and elimination are relatively slower than in the mother. Carbon monoxide interferes with tissue oxygenation and therefore has potentially damaging effects on the fetus. Theoretically, even short periods of exposure may interfere with embryonic or fetal development. Longo suggests that maternal smoking, by resulting in higher than normal carbon monoxide levels in the mother and the fetus may be the cause of impaired growth. However, it must be said that there is still uncertainty about the mechanism between adverse outcome for the fetus and smoking in pregnancy.

## The effects of nicotine on the uteroplacental vasculature as vasoconstrictor

Animal studies have been performed to try and elucidate the mechanism by which other substances derived from smoking might have adverse effects on the outcome of pregnancy.

In attempting to address the multifactorial content of the influence of smoking in pregnancy outcome, Becker et al. (1968) injected female Osborne–Mendel rats with either normal saline twice daily or with nicotine in doses of 0.5, 1.0, 3.0, and 5.0 mg per kilogram body weight, and compared the outcome with an untreated control population. The injections caused behavioural changes in the maternal rat with circling, tremor, mild convulsions, severe convulsions, and apnoeic episodes at the higher levels of nicotine, even though the higher doses were considered to be far below the $LD_{50}$ for this species.

Maternal food consumption and weight gain were recorded and maternal weight was recorded on a weekly basis throughout pregnancy. These investigators demonstrated that the higher the dosage of nicotine administered, the less the amount of food eaten in the first week of pregnancy. Thereafter, all animals gained weight at the same rate. Overall, the animals receiving nicotine exhibited lower weight gain.

Mothers receiving high doses of nicotine delivered significantly fewer live born per litter and the young weighed significantly less than the control population. Furthermore, of the animals born alive in the high nicotine dosage group, fewer animals survived the first week after delivery.

Clearly, there are limits to the conclusions that can be reached from these data, as they do not preclude the effects of the changes induced on nutritional status or the effect of pregnant convulsions induced by nicotine, which are not part of the observed effects in human smoking. None of these data point specifically to a direct impairment of placental infusion by a vasoconstrictor effect on the uterine vasculature, but such an effect cannot be excluded.

Tomasi et al. (1987) studied the haemodynamic response in the dams to continuous intravenous infusion using two different infusion rates and radiolabelled microspheres in pregnant guinea pigs. The infusion of a low-dose nicotine at 4.5 µg/min had no significant effect on cardiac output or uteroplacental blood flow, but during high dose infusion at 18 µg/min produced a significant fall in both cardiac output and uteroplacental blood flow.

Blood levels of nicotine were measured and, at levels two to five times greater than those seen in smokers, there were no measurable effects.

Monheit *et al.* (1983) examined the effect of nicotine on uterine and umbilical haemodynamics in seven pregnant ewes. In this study, electromagnetic flow probes were used to measure flow in the main uterine and umbilical vessels. As with the guinea pig studies, high dosage infusion rates of 1.0–1.5 mg/min reduce uterine and umbilical blood flow by 42 and 32 per cent respectively. However, infusion rates of 0.5 mg/min, which, in themselves, resulted in mean peak maternal nicotine concentrations of $130 \pm 5.0$ mg/ml, a value substantially higher than that found in human cigarette smokers, did not significantly alter uterine or umbilical vascular haemodynamics. The lower infusion rates also failed to produce any change in maternal or fetal catecholamine levels.

These studies indicate that smoking is unlikely to produce any detrimental effects in terms of oxygen transfer by reducing blood flow to the vascular beds related to oxygen transfer to the fetus.

## Conclusions

1. Cigarette smoke contains high concentrations of carbon monoxide and therefore carries a significant risk to maternal and fetal well-being.
2. Carbon monoxide shifts the oxygen dissociation curve to the left in both maternal and fetal blood and therefore may interfere with tissue oxygen delivery in the fetus and placenta.
3. Carbon monoxide saturation may rise to 7.6 per cent in the fetus and 8.3 per cent in the mother in cigarette smokers. These changes are particularly likely to be significant where the uteroplacental blood flow is already impaired.
4. Carbon monoxide uptake and elimination is relatively slower in the mother than the fetus.
5. The effect of nicotine on the uterine circulation is unlikely to be a factor in contributing to any impairment of oxygen transfer.

## References

Asmussen, I. and Kjeldsen, K. (1975). Intimal ultrastructure of human umbilical arteries. Observations on arteries from newborn children of smoking and nonsmoking mothers. *Circulation Research*, **36**, 579–83.

Becker, R. F., Little, C. R. D., and King, J. E. (1968). Experimental studies on nicotine absorption in rats during pregnancy: III. Effect of subcutaneous injection of small chronic doses upon mother, fetus and neonate. *American Journal of Obstetrics and Gynecology*, **100(7)**, 957–68.

Begley, D. J., Firth, J. A., and Hoult, J. R. S. (1980). In *Human reproduction and developmental biology*, pp. 78. Ch. 7 The Placenta. The MacMillan Press Ltd, London.

Douglas, C. G., Haldane, J. S., and Haldane, J. B. S. (1912). The laws of combination of hemoglobin with carbon monoxide and oxygen. *Journal of Physiology (Lond)*, **44**, 275–9.

Gennser, G., Marsal, K., and Brantmark, B. (1975). Maternal smoking and fetal breathing movements. *American Journal of Obstetrics and Gynecology*, **123(8)**, 861–7.

Longo, L. D. (1977). The biological effects of carbon monoxide on the pregnant woman, fetus and newborn infant. *American Journal of Obstetrics and Gynecology*, **129**, 69–103.

Longo, L. D. and Hill, E. P. (1977). Carbon monoxide uptake and elimination in fetal and maternal sheep. *American Journal of Physiology*, **232**, H324.

Meyer, M. B. and Comstock, G. W. (1972). Maternal cigarette smoking and perinatal mortality. *American Journal of Epidemiology*, **96**, 1–3.

Miller, H. C. and Hassanein, K. (1974). Maternal smoking and fetal growth of full term infants. *Pediatric Research*, **8**, 960–3.

Monheit, A. G., VanVunakis, H., Key, T. C., and Resnik, R. (1983). Maternal and fetal cardiovascular effects of nicotine infusion in pregnant sheep. *American Journal of Obstetrics and Gynecology*, **145(3)**, 290–4.

Robinson, S. and Robbins, R. C. (1970). Atmospheric background concentrations of carbon monoxide. *Annals of the New York Academy of Sciences*, **174**, 89–93.

Roughton, F. J. W. and Darling, R. C. (1944). The effect of carbon monoxide on the oxyhemoglobin dissociation curve. *American Journal of Physiology*, **141**, 17–19.

Tomasi, A. M., Lee, H., and Myers, S. (1987). The hemodynamic response of the conscious pregnant guinea pig to nicotine. *American Journal of Obstetrics and Gynecology*, **156(4)**, 1015–18.

# 7. Smoking and pre-eclampsia

*Marion H Hall and Valerie Harper*

## Introduction

A substantially lower incidence of hypertensive complications of pregnancy in cigarette smoking was shown 20–30 years ago in some large hospital-based studies (Underwood *et al*. 1965; Duffus and MacGillivray 1968; Kullander and Kallen 1972; Palmgren *et al*. 1973) although this was not found in the first study to look at the topic (Zabriskie 1963). Community-based studies (Butler and Alberman 1969; Andrews and McGarry 1972; Chamberlain *et al*. 1978) subsequently confirmed the phenomenon, and some recent case-control studies (Ounsted and Scott 1982; Moore and Redman 1983; Marcoux *et al*. 1989) again identified the association. The effect is dose-dependent (Kullander and Kallen 1972; Palmgren *et al*. 1979; Chamberlain *et al*. 1978; Marcoux *et al*. 1989), suggesting it may be causally related to maternal smoking. However, many different definitions of pre-eclampsia were used, making it difficult to assess whether the effect is on gestational hypertension or on pre-eclampsia, as defined by international agreement (Davey and MacGillivray 1986). Smoking habit was recorded after delivery in most studies, with possible ascertainment bias.

The apparently beneficial effect of smoking on pre-eclampsia was mitigated by reports of higher perinatal mortality in the smokers who did develop pre-eclampsia. In the early 1960s, when perinatal mortality rates were much higher than now, perinatal death was 2.6 times more common in a group of pre-eclamptic mothers who smoked compared to those who did not (Duffus and MacGillivray 1968). However, only ten deaths were involved, and the perinatal mortality due to hypertension in the whole group of smokers was not significantly higher than in the non-smokers. In the 1970 British Births Survey (Chamberlain *et al*. 1978) perinatal mortality was 2.3 times higher in 457 women with pre-eclampsia who smoked than in 402 who did not. The 33 deaths were not categorized by cause of death. Among 2928 women with hypertension in Wales (Andrews and McGarry 1972), smokers had a perinatal mortality rate of 5.1 per cent compared to 3.1 per cent in non-smokers. The 111 deaths were not classified by cause. The contribution of smoking is, therefore, difficult to assess.

Possible mechanisms for the findings in pre-eclampsia are:

1. Smoking is associated with poor maternal weight gain (Underwood *et al*.

1965; Rush 1974) and pre-eclampsia with high weight gain (MacGillivray 1961). However, as high weight gain is unlikely to be the cause of pre-eclampsia, it is not surprising that the association of pre-eclampsia with smoking is at least partly independent of weight gain (Duffus and MacGillivray 1968; Andrews and McGarry 1972).

2. That smoking may cause either first trimester abortion or pre-eclampsia, and that the deficit in pre-eclampsia may be attributable to prior spontaneous abortion (Palmgren *et al.* 1973). However, Kullander and Kallen (1972) found no increase in first trimester abortion, but only in late abortion, especially when pregnancy was unwanted and abortion may have been induced. The topic of the possible effect of smoking on spontaneous abortion has not often been studied in the same population as births.

3. An increase amongst smokers in a cyanide detoxification product (thiocyanate) may have an anti-hypertensive effect (Andrews and McGarry 1972).

4. Nicotine may inhibit thromboxane $A_2$ synthesis in fetal platelets (Ylikorkola *et al.* 1985) and modify the maternal level, which is usually increased in pre-eclampsia (Wallenburg and Potmans 1982).

Whatever the mechanism, it remains to be seen what the effect on pre-eclampsia is of anti-smoking education, and the effect on its severity of modern methods of screening and antenatal, intrapartum and neonatal management. Using recent population-based data from the Aberdeen Maternity and Neonatal Databank, we have re-examined the association between smoking and pre-eclampsia, and the association of smoking with perinatal mortality, extended perinatal mortality, and birth weight for gestational age, in all women and in those with pre-eclampsia.

## Methods

The 28 563 singleton deliveries between 1980 and 1989 of all women resident in Aberdeen City District were analysed. The geographical area is identical to that used by Duffus and MacGillivray (1968), but no exclusions on the grounds of multiparity, booking or marital status were made. Number of cigarettes smoked was recorded prospectively, and women who stopped smoking early in pregnancy were categorized as non-smokers. Hypertension in pregnancy was defined as recommended by Davey and MacGillivray (1986). Classification of cause of perinatal death was according to the modified Baird classification (Cole *et al.* 1986). 'Extended perinatal mortality' includes deaths from 24 weeks gestation until the end of the first 4 weeks of life. Birth weight for gestational age was analysed using locally derived centile distributions corrected for gestational age, parity and babies' sex. These are available from 32 weeks for male babies and from 33 weeks for females.

# Results

## Pre-eclampsia

Among 28 563 singleton births, 10 623 women (37.2 per cent) smoked. The rate of smoking was identical in primigravidae and parous women. Of the 4910 primigravidae who smoked, 258 (5.3 per cent), and in the 8295 non-smokers 662 (8.0 per cent), had pre-eclampsia. There was a similar difference of incidence in the parous women, 94 (1.6 per cent) of the 5713 parous women who smoked, and 247 (2.6 per cent) of the 9641 non-smokers had pre-eclampsia. Gestational hypertension was also reduced in the smokers by a similar amount: 1137 (23.2 per cent) of primigravidae who smoked and 2477 (29.9 per cent) of non-smoking primigravidae had gestational hypertension. In the parous women gestational hypertension was present in 630 (11.0 per cent) of the smokers and 87 (15.4 per cent) of the non-smokers. There was no gradient in the incidence of pre-eclampsia with the number of cigarettes smoked per day (Table 7.1). The mean age of the smokers was 24.9 years, compared with 26.9 years in the non-smokers. Because pre-eclampsia is more common in older women an analysis was done to see whether the younger age of the smokers explained this lower incidence of pre-eclampsia. Table 7.2 shows that in each age group the incidence of pre-eclampsia is lower in smokers than in non-smokers with the exception of the 84 smoking primigravidae aged 35 years or more, of whom 13 (15.5 per cent) had pre-eclampsia. However, these numbers are small and the data do not support younger age as an explanation for the effect of smoking on pre-eclampsia.

## Perinatal mortality

Considering perinatal deaths in all women (Table 7.3) the expected higher rate in smokers is evident for all causes of death, for death excluding lethal congenital malformation, and for deaths due to causes that might be attribut-

**Table 7.1** Incidence of pre-eclampsia by number of cigarettes smoked per day: singletons 1980–1989

| Number smoked | Primigravidae | | | Parity 1+ | | |
|---|---|---|---|---|---|---|
| | Total | Pre-eclampsia | | Total | Pre-eclampsia | |
| | | *n* | % | | *n* | % |
| 1–9 | 918 | 47 | 5.1 | 744 | 13 | 1.7 |
| 10–19 | 2170 | 109 | 5.0 | 2543 | 42 | 1.7 |
| 20 | 1203 | 55 | 4.6 | 1996 | 34 | 1.7 |

**Table 7.2** Percentage incidence of pre-eclampsia by age, parity and smoking: singleton 1980–1989

| Age | Primigravidae | | Parity 1+ | |
|---|---|---|---|---|
| | Non-smokers ($n = 8299$) | Smokers ($n = 4910$) | Non-smokers ($n = 9641$) | Smokers ($n = 5713$) |
| ≤ 19 | 8.7 | 4.7 | 2.6 | 0.5 |
| 20–34 | 7.9 | 5.1 | 2.5 | 1.6 |
| 35+ | 9.2 | 15.5 | 3.2 | 3.0 |

**Table 7.3** Perinatal mortality by selected cause and maternal smoking: singletons 1980–1989

| | Non-smokers ($n = 17940$) | | Smokers ($n = 10653$) | |
|---|---|---|---|---|
| | $n$ | rate/000 | $n$ | rate/000 |
| All perinatal deaths | 150 | 8.4 | 117 | 11.0 |
| All deaths except congenital malformation | 105 | 5.5 | 92 | 8.7 |
| Deaths due to antepartum or intrapartum asphyxia, abruption, pre-eclampsia or maternal disease | 69 | 3.8 | 64 | 6.0 |
| Deaths due to pre-eclampsia | 7 | 0.4 | 5 | 0.5 |

able to smoking (antepartum or intrapartum asphyxia, abruption, pre-eclampsia or maternal disease). Only when looking at deaths due to pre-eclampsia alone is there no difference, and numbers are very small.

Looking at perinatal mortality in cases of pre-eclampsia (Table 7.4) there is no difference between smokers and non-smokers. However, using extended perinatal mortality from 24 weeks until 4 weeks of age, the death rate is twice as great in the smokers ($z = 2.025$; $P < 0.05$).

## Birthweight for gestation

Average gestation length in smokers with pre-eclampsia was shorter (at 37.8 weeks) than in non-smokers (38.2 weeks). Average birth weight in smokers with pre-eclampsia was less (at 2875 g) than in non-smokers (3030 g). The

**Table 7.4** Perinatal mortality in women with pre-eclampsia by smoking: singleton births 1980–1989

|                                          | Non-smokers ($n = 909$) | | Smokers ($n = 352$) | |
|------------------------------------------|-------|--------|-------|--------|
| Spontaneous abortions                    | 2     |        | 7     |        |
| Stillbirths                              | 11    |        | 6     |        |
| First week deaths                        | 4     |        | 0     |        |
| First month deaths                       | 1     |        | 1     |        |
| Total perinatal deaths (rate/000)        | 15    | (16.5) | 6     | (17.0) |
| Extended perinatal deaths (rate/000)     | 18    | (19.8) | 14    | (39.8) |

**Table 7.5** Birth weight centile distributions (corrected for gestational age, parity and babies' sex) by smoking and pre-eclampsia: singleton births 1980–1989

| Centiles        | All women ($n = 28\,509$) | Non-smokers ($n = 17\,904$) | Smokers ($n\ 10\,605$) | Pre-eclampsia ($n = 1260$) | Pre-eclampsia | |
|-----------------|------|------|------|------|---------------------------------|------------------------|
|                 |      |      |      |      | Non-smokers ($n = 908$) | Smokers ($n = 352$) |
| Not classified* | 1.9  | 1.6  | 2.4  | 4.3  | 3.3  | 6.8  |
| $\leq$ 5th      | 4.4  | 2.6  | 7.4  | 6.7  | 6.2  | 7.9  |
| > 5th $\geqq$ 10th | 4.7 | 3.2 | 7.1 | 7.1 | 6.5 | 8.5 |
| > 10th < 90th   | 78.2 | 79.4 | 76.1 | 70.8 | 72.3 | 66.8 |
| $\leq$ 90th < 95th | 5.5 | 6.7 | 3.7 | 5.5 | 6.1 | 4.3 |
| $\leq$ 95th     | 5.3  | 6.5  | 3.3  | 5.6  | 5.6  | 5.7  |

* Cases are not classified if data items are missing or if gestational age is less than 33 weeks in girls and 32 weeks in boys.

distribution of birth weight centiles corrected for gestation, parity, and babies' sex, is shown in Table 7.5.

As expected, smoking is associated with reduced birth weight across the whole range of weight, while in pre-eclampsia there are more babies (13.5 per cent) less than the 10th centile, but no reduction in the proportion greater than the 90th centile. The combination of smoking and pre-eclampsia has a particularly severe effect on smaller babies, with 16.4 per cent less than the 10th centile, but very little difference in the proportion greater than the 90th centile. The differences between non-smokers and smokers in the women with pre-eclampsia is significant ($\chi^2 = 12.59$; $P < 0.05$).

Table 7.6 shows that in the deliveries before 33 weeks, although the

**Table 7.6** Distribution of gestation and average birth weight in women delivering from 24–32 weeks by pre-eclampsia and smoking: singletons 1980–1989

| Gestation at delivery (weeks) | All women | | Pre-eclampsia | | Pre-eclampsia and smoking | |
|---|---|---|---|---|---|---|
| | *n* | % | *n* | % | *n* | % |
| 24–27 | 116 | 26.5 | 12 | 19.7 | 8 | 30.8 |
| 28–29 | 93 | 21.3 | 15 | 24.6 | 5 | 19.2 |
| 30–32 | 220 | 52.2 | 39 | 55.7 | 13 | 50.0 |
| Total | 437 | 100.0 | 61 | 100.0 | 26 | 100.0 |
| Average birth weight (g) | 1335 | | 1156 | | 996 | |

distribution of gestational age at delivery was not significantly different, average birth weight was reduced in women with pre-eclampsia, and further reduced in women who smoked. Both reductions were significant ($P < 0.05$).

## Discussion

Taking account of recent education of pregnant women about smoking, it is surprising that the smoking rate in this population is similar to that documented in the early 1960s. However, the earlier study was confined to booked married women, whereas these restrictions are not considered appropriate now, so there may be a real reduction in smoking. The difference in the pre-eclampsia rate between smokers and non-smokers is very similar to that in the earlier study. The actual pre-eclampsia rate in primigravidae is higher now than in the earlier study, perhaps because of better ascertainment. The absence of a clear dose–response gradient by number of cigarettes smoked might cast doubt upon whether the association of smoking with less pre-eclampsia is a causal one. However, the lower pre-eclampsia rate in smokers is not attributable to other maternal characteristics, such as primigravidity or older age.

Perintal death due to pre-eclampsia constitutes only a small proportion of overall perinatal deaths, and is not more common in smokers, though most other causes are. The perinatal death rate in women with pre-eclampsia is so much lower now that numbers are small but, looking at extended perinatal mortality, and taking into account the earlier age of viability and increased neonatal survival, there is still a higher death rate in the babies of smokers who develop pre-eclampsia than in non-smokers. Most of the excess deaths are very early, but throughout the range of gestational age there is evidence of disadvantage in the smokers in that birth weight for gestational age is reduced. There is, therefore, no justification for considering the lower pre-eclampsia rate in smokers as an advantage, and there should be no hesitation in discouraging smoking in pregnancy.

## Acknowledgements

We would like to thank Dr Doris Campbell and Mr John Lemon for computing assistance and advice. Valerie Harper is funded by the Scottish Home and Health Department.

## References

Andrews, S. and McGarry, J. M. (1972). A community study of smoking in pregnancy. *Journal of Obstetrics and Gynaecology of the British Commonwealth,* **79,** 1057–73.

Butler, N. R. and Alberman, E. D. (1969). High risk predictors at booking and in pregnancy. In *Perinatal problems.* The Second Report of the 1958 British Perinatal Mortality Survey, pp. 36–46. E & S Livingstone Ltd., Edinburgh.

Chamberlain, G., Philipp, E., Howlett, B., and Masters, K. (1978). *Hypertension in British births 1970, vol. 2, obstetric care,* pp. 80–107. Heinemann, London.

Cole, S. K., Hey, E. N., and Thomson, A. M. (1986). Classifying perinatal death: An obstetric approach. *British Journal of Obstetrics and Gynaecology,* **93,** 1204–12.

Davey, D. A. and MacGillivray, I. (1986). The classification and definition of hypertensive disorders of pregnancy. *Clinical Experimental Hypertension (Basel),* **5,** 97–133.

Duffus, G. M. and MacGillivray, I. (1968). The incidence of pre-eclamptic toxaemia in smokers and non-smokers. *Lancet,* **i,** 994–5.

Kullander, S. and Kallen, B. (1972). A prospective study of smoking and pregnancy. *Acta Obstetricia Gynecologicia Scandinavica,* **50,** 83–94.

MacGillivray, I. (1961). Hypertension and its consequences. *Journal of Obstetrics and Gynaecology of the British Commonwealth,* **68,** 557–69.

Marcoux, S., Brisson, J., and Fabia, J. (1989). The effect of cigarette smoking on the risk of pre-eclampsia and gestational hypertension. *American Journal of Epidemiology,* **130,** 950–7.

Moore, M. P. and Redman, C. W. G. (1983). Case control study of severe pre-eclampsia of early onset. *British Medical Journal,* **287,** 580–3.

Ounsted, M. and Scott, A. (1982). Smoking during pregnancy in association with other maternal factors and birthweight. *Acta Obstetricia Gynecologicia Scandinavica,* **61,** 367–71.

Palmgren, B., Wahlen, T., and Wallonder, B. (1973). Toxaemia and cigarette smoking during pregnancy. Prospective consecutive investigation of 3927 pregnancies. *Acta Obstetricia Gynecologicia Scandinavica,* **52,** 183–5.

Rush, D. (1974). Examination of the relationship between birthweight, cigarette smoking during pregnancy and maternal weight gain. *Journal of Obstetrics and Gynaecology of the British Commonwealth,* **81,** 746–52.

Underwood, P. B., Hestler, L. L., Lafitte, T. Jr, and Gregg, K. V. (1965). The relationship of smoking to the outcome of pregnancy. *American Journal of Obstetrics and Gynecology,* **91,** 270–6.

Wallenburg, H. C. S. and Potmans, N. (1982). Enhanced reactivity of the platelet thromboxane pathway in normotensive and hypertensive pregnancies with insufficient fetal growth. *American Journal of Obstetrics and Gynecology,* **144,** 523–7.

Ylikorkola, O, Viinikka, L., and Lehtovirta, P. (1985). Effect of nicotine on fetal prostacyclin and thromboxane in humans. *Obstetrics and Gynecology,* **66,** 102–5.

Zabriskie, J. R. (1963). Effect of cigarette smoking during pregnancy. *Obstetrics and Gynecology,* **21,** 405–11.

# 8. The effects of smoking on fetal growth: evidence for a threshold, the importance of brand of cigarette, and interaction with alcohol and caffeine consumption

*H Ross Anderson, J Martin Bland, and Janet L Peacock*

## Introduction

The achievement of optimum fetal growth is accepted as a desirable clinical and public health objective. In so far as perinatal mortality and morbidity, with their attendant personal, social, and economic costs are increased as the birth weight distribution is shifted downwards, the reduction in fetal growth (birth weight adjusted for gestational age) observed with smoking, while clinically unimportant for most pregnancies, is of considerable public health importance (US Department of Health and Human Services 1980; Dunn 1984; Oster *et al.* 1988).

The association between cigarette smoking and reduced birth weight has been known for some time (Simpson 1957; Andrews and McGarry 1972; Butler *et al.* 1972; US Department of Health and Human Services 1980; McIntosh 1984). Some have suggested that this is not causal but explained by other factors, such as diet, personal characteristics, or psychosocial stress, which may relate to both fetal growth and smoking behaviour (Yerushalmy 1971; Rush and Cassano 1983). Most authorities, however, have concluded that the association is causal because it is found in a wide variety of study designs and epidemiological contexts, exhibits a dose–response relationship, and has biological plausibility (Abel 1980; US Department of Health and Human Services 1980). A causal relationship is also suggested by the usual finding that smokers who give up at any time before 30 weeks have heavier infants than persistent smokers (MacArthur and Knox 1988).

The mechanism by which smoking exerts an effect on birth weight is unclear. One possibility is that one or more of the many constituents of tobacco smoke may influence fetal growth by direct toxicity. Another is that the effects may be more indirect through damage to or functional disturbance of the placenta. Smoking might also affect birth weight indirectly by influencing appetite, nutritional intake, and maternal metabolism (Picone *et al.* 1982), but most authorities consider this to be a less likely mechanism in a well nourished population (US Department of Health and Human Services 1980). Animal studies have shown that at least two important constituents of cigarette smoke—carbon monoxide and nicotine—have detrimental effects on the fetus (US Department of Health and Human Services 1980, 1981).

A number of aspects of the relationship between smoking and fetal growth require further exploration. These include the role of smoking in mediating or interacting with other potential hazards, such as psychosocial stress, poor diet, and other behaviours, especially consumption of alcohol and caffeine in pregnancy. Another relatively unexplored area in epidemiological studies is the nature and mechanism of the relationship between smoking and fetal growth and, in particular the relative importance of the various constituents, the number of cigarettes smoked and the gestational age of exposure.

The St George's Birthweight Study was set up to investigate these, among other, questions. It was intended to bridge the gap that exists between very large studies, which tend, of necessity, to be thin on detail, narrow in scope, and variable in the quality of measures of exposure and outcome, and small studies, which though sometimes strong on detail inevitably suffer the disadvantage of being weak in statistical power. This chapter will bring together both published (Brooke et al. 1989; Peacock 1989; Peacock et al. 1991) and unpublished data from the St George's Birthweight Study in an attempt to shed light on the following aspects of the problem:

1. The effect of smoking on fetal growth, including the relationship with quantity of cigarettes smoked, yield of brand of cigarette smoked, and gestational age of exposure.
2. Interactions between smoking and consumption of alcohol and caffeine.
3. The need for the above analyses to control for possible confounding by psychosocial factors.

## Methods

At St George's Hospital, which serves the inner London teaching Health District of Wandsworth, 1860 consecutive white women were invited to take part in a study of factors affecting birth weight. The target sample size was 1500, this being calculated as being sufficient to show with high power significant differences between subgroups (as small as 10 per cent of the total) of 180 g, the anticipated difference in birth weight between smokers and non-smokers. Interviews were conducted in private by trained research interviewers at booking (mean 14 weeks), 3 weeks after booking (mean 17 weeks), and at 28 and 36 weeks gestation.

Data were obtained about marital state (both civil and 'effective'), education, employment, tenure, household structure, amenities, and income. Anxiety and depression were measured on three occasions using the 28-item general health questionnaire (Goldberg and Hillier 1979) and stressful life events were recorded using the interview developed by Paykel (Paykel *et al.* 1969). Various other measures of satisfaction with social, personal, and environmental circumstances were obtained. Social support, receipt of state benefits and the attitude to pregnancy were assessed.

Data on smoking and the consumption of alcohol and caffeine containing drinks were obtained at booking, 28, and 36 weeks and pertained to consumption in the week before interview. Information about previous smoking, inhalation habit, and exposure to smoke of others in the household was obtained at booking only. The brand smoked was recorded at each interview. From the brand given, the tar, nicotine, and carbon monoxide yields were recorded using the analysis of the Government Chemist (UK Department of Health 1983). Smoking was validated in a subsample using plasma thiocyanate estimations. Alcohol intake was determined from the type of drink consumed and its quantity (in pub measures) and converted into grams of alcohol using a standard method (Paul and Southgate 1978). Total caffeine consumption for each week was estimated using estimates of for tea (70 mg/cup) and coffee (92 mg/cup) from a UK study (Al-Samarrae *et al.* 1975), and for cocoa (5 mg/cup) and cola (40 mg/serving) from another report (Graham 1978).

Obstetric data were obtained from the structured obstetric record. Birth weight was measured by a midwife within 30 min of birth with a spring balance (Marsden, London). Gestational age at delivery was calculated from the date of delivery recorded by the obstetrician based on dates of menstruation and results of early ultrasound examination (routine at the time of this survey). The outcome variable for the present analysis was fetal growth, this being inferred from birth weight adjusted for gestational age. Adjustment was done by taking the ratio of the observed birth weight to that expected for the gestational age using an external standard (Keen and Pearse 1985). The statistical rationale and method is described in detail elsewhere (Bland *et al.* 1990). Once adjusted for gestational age the ratio was then adjusted for maternal height, sex of infant, and parity using multiple regression. The mother's age was not included because it had no independent effect. This method gave an adjusted birth weight ratio (ABWR), which was suitable for analysis using least squares regression. All the mean ABWRs were close to 1.00, which means that the difference between two ratios was equivalent to a proportional difference, e.g. 1.04 and 0.99 differ by 0.05, or by 5 per cent. Additional descriptions of statistical methods used for analysing quantity and yield of cigarettes are included in the results section where appropriate, but details may also be found in published reports (Peacock 1989; Peacock *et al.* 1991). As some questionnaires had missing data the total numbers in the different tables are subject to variation.

## Results

Of the 1860 women invited to enter the study, 1513 (81 per cent) completed the interviews at booking and 3 weeks later at 17 weeks. Losses were due to refusal to participate at the outset (136), spontaneous abortion (53), change of address (54), missing data on important biological variables (26), and missed interviews (56). Twenty-two women with either macerated stillbirth or major congenital malformation were excluded. The number with completed interviews up to 28 weeks was 1463 and up to 36 weeks was 1433. Some of these did not have adequate smoking data and the numbers that form the basis of the present analyses are: booking, 1513; 28 weeks, 1414; and 36 weeks, 1400.

The distribution of smoking habit at each interview is shown in Table 8.1. About 30 per cent were smoking at each interview and of these the proportion smoking 15 or more cigarettes per day was 31 per cent at booking, rising to 36 per cent at 28 and 36 weeks. Mean consumption was 11.1, 12.1, and 11.7 cigarettes per day for the respective interviews. Of those for whom brand data were available, a minority smoked low tar (20–25 per cent) with about equal proportions smoking low to middle tar (36–38 per cent) or middle tar (39–43 per cent). Of the 1309 for whom a full smoking history, including brand smoked, was available on each occasion, 340 reported smoking at each interview (consistent smokers), 74 at only one or two interviews, and 895 were not smoking at any interview.

At each interview, the mean serum thiocyanate levels of non-smokers was

**Table 8.1** Distribution of smoking at each interview

|  | Booking | | 28 weeks | | 36 weeks | |
|---|---|---|---|---|---|---|
|  | $n = 1513$ | % | $n = 1414$ | % | $n = 1400$ | % |
| Non-smokers | 1022 | 68 | 965 | 68 | 975 | 70 |
| (never smoked) | (400) | | | | | |
| (Ex before preg) | (492) | | | | | |
| (Ex in this preg) | (130) | | | | | |
| Smokers | 491 | 32 | 449 | 32 | 425 | 30 |
| 1–4 | 117 | | 97 | | 96 | |
| 5–9 | 101 | | 92 | | 78 | |
| 10–14 | 118 | | 100 | | 99 | |
| 15–19 | 63 | | 72 | | 59 | |
| 20–29 | 77 | | 69 | | 78 | |
| 30+ | 14 | | 19 | | 15 | |
|  | $n = 459*$ | | $n = 425*$ | | $n = 400*$ | |
| Low tar | 94 | 20 | 93 | 22 | 98 | 25 |
| Low to middle tar | 165 | 36 | 160 | 38 | 145 | 36 |
| Middle tar | 199 | 43 | 172 | 40 | 157 | 39 |
| Middle to high | 1 | | 0 | | 0 | |

* Reduced number of subjects because of missing histories.

between 30 and 31 μmol/l. This was significantly less than the levels of between 63 and 74 μmol/l observed in the smokers.

The effects of smoking on ABWR are shown in Table 8.2 for smoking recorded at each interview. Amongst non-smokers there was virtually no difference in birth weight between never smokers and ex-smokers, whether they had quit before pregnancy or in early pregnancy. For the assessment at booking, the birth weight of smokers was 4.9 per cent below that of non-smokers (equivalent to −171 g at term), with similar decrements observed at 28 and 36 weeks. When the smokers were divided by number of cigarettes smoked into < 15/day and 15+/day, the babies of heavier smokers were 2–3 per cent smaller than those of light smokers. Among non-smokers, those who were exposed passively to the smoke of others had babies with weights 0.05 per cent lower than non-exposed mothers (equivalent to 18 g at term; $P = 0.56$).

The association between ABWR and alcohol consumption at each interview

**Table 8.2** Mean adjusted birth weight ratio and smoking habit reported at 14, 28, and 36 weeks

| Smoking habit | Number* | ABWR | BW adjusted to 40 weeks† | Test of significance | |
|---|---|---|---|---|---|
| **Booking** | | | | | |
| Non-smokers | 1022 | 1.053 | 3675 | Non-smokers versus smokers | $P < 0.01$ |
| Never smoked | 400 | 1.054 | 3678 | Never smokers versus ex-smokers | $P = 0.78$ |
| Ex pre-pregnancy | 492 | 1.052 | 3671 | | |
| Ex early pregnancy | 130 | 1.052 | 3671 | | |
| Smokers | 491 | 1.004 | 3504 | | |
| 1–14/day | 336 | 1.013 | 3535 | 1–14 versus 15+ | $P = 0.02$ |
| 15+/day | 154 | 0.984 | 3434 | | |
| **28 weeks** | | | | | |
| Non-smokers | 965 | 1.052 | 3671 | Non-smokers versus smokers | $P < 0.001$ |
| Smokers | 449 | 1.002 | 3497 | | |
| 1–14/day | 289 | 1.012 | 3532 | 1–14 versus 15+ | $P = 0.02$ |
| 15+/day | 160 | 0.984 | 3434 | | |
| **36 weeks** | | | | | |
| Non-smokers | 975 | 1.050 | 3664 | Non-smokers versus smokers | $P < 0.001$ |
| Smokers | 425 | 0.998 | 3486 | | |
| 1–14/day | 273 | 1.007 | 3514 | 1–14 versus 15+ | $P = 0.06$ |
| 15+/day | 152 | 0.984 | 3434 | | |

* Reduced number of subjects due to missing histories.
† Adjusted to 40 weeks gestation, male child, maternal height 160 cm, parity 1+.
ABWR, adjusted birth weight ratio; BW, birth weight.

is shown in Table 8.3. At booking, 50 per cent of women reported drinking alcohol in the previous week. There was a significant trend towards lower birth weight as consumption increased. The difference between non-drinkers and heavy drinkers (100 g/week) was 4 per cent—equivalent to 137 g at term. Similar relationships were observed at 28 and 36 weeks, though the trends were not significant. We already knew that smokers in our sample were more likely to drink alcohol (Heller *et al.* 1988) and therefore analysed the effects of alcohol within smoking categories (Table 8.3). Within non-smokers there was no evidence of an association between alcohol and birth weight and, if anything, the trend was towards higher birth weight with increased drinking. Among smokers, however, there was a clear and significant trend towards lower birth weight with increased drinking. Non-drinking smokers had a mean birth weight that was 7 per cent higher (equivalent to 241 g at term) than smokers who drank more than 100 g/w. Within the smoking group, multiple regression of ABWR on numbers of cigarettes and alcohol found that each effect remained significant while controlling for the other.

Separate analyses were done for tea, coffee, cola, and total caffeine consumption. At booking, consumption of tea and coffee, but not cola, was significantly associated with reduced birth weight. These associations tended to become weaker at 28 and 36 weeks. Total caffeine intake was estimated and a significant trend was observed. As for alcohol, the analyses were repeated after dividing by smoking status because consumption is positively related to smoking. It was found that while among non-smokers there was no trend in birth weight with consumption, among smokers, there were downward trends in birth weight with tea, coffee, and total caffeine. The effects of smoking on birth weight remained significant after controlling for these consumptions. Among smokers, multiple regression of birth weight on number of cigarettes and caffeine showed that both had independent effects.

In examining the effect of smoking on fetal growth retardation, other factors that needed to be considered were those that could be categorized as psychosocial and socio-economic. These might act directly by influencing hormonal or even neural mechanisms that affect fetal growth. Alternatively, they might act through associations with factors such as impaired maternal growth (reduced height, for example), or detrimental behaviours (smoking, alcohol, poor diet). The factors examined have been outlined in the methods section and their associations with birth weight have been reported in detail elsewhere (Brooke *et al.* 1989). Out of over 40 indicators examined, only five were found to be associated with reduced birth weight. These were:

(1) missed antenatal visits;
(2) manual social class (only when based on the mother's occupation);
(3) mother's employer knowing that she was pregnant;
(4) lower school leaving age;
(5) help with fares to hospital.

All these effects disappeared after smoking was controlled for, while controlling for these factors did not remove the significant effect of smoking. Based on the results of this analysis, there was justification for ignoring the possible confounding effects of these factors in the analyses of the effects of smoking, alcohol, and caffeine on ABWR.

It was now established that, after controlling for 'biological' variables (parity, maternal height, sex of child), the main factors measured in the study affecting fetal growth were smoking and, amongst smokers only, alcohol and caffeine consumption. The interaction between smoking and alcohol and caffeine needed to be explored further but before this could be done, it was necessary to obtain a better understanding of the relationship between the quantity smoked and birth weight, so that smoking could be adequately controlled in the analysis. Also of interest was the effect of brand of cigarette, as well as which constituents of tobacco smoke might be important, and when.

Linear regression of ABWR on numbers of cigarettes smoked and the yields of the brands smoked was performed and the results of this are shown in Table 8.4 for the week 28 interview for those who were consistent smokers (smoking at each interview). When analysed separately, both the number smoked and carbon monoxide yield of the brand were negatively related to ABWR. The relationship with carbon monoxide was stronger than that with the number of cigarettes as shown by the proportion of variability explained (Table 8.4; $R^2$). When both carbon monoxide and number of cigarettes were included in the model, both had significant effects on ABWR. When an interaction term was added, this was not significant, although it was positive, suggesting that the effect on ABWR of the number of cigarettes was greater for smokers of low-yield cigarettes than for smokers of high-yield cigarettes. As Table 8.4 shows, very similar results were obtained when carbon monoxide was replaced by tar or nicotine.

The intercorrelations between tar, nicotine, and carbon monoxide were very strong ($r = 0.93$, $0.96$, and $0.97$, respectively) making it impossible to estimate their independent effects if any. Therefore analyses using carbon monoxide are presented in the rest of this chapter. Results for tar and nicotine were very similar.

The analysis described above was also done for the booking and week 36 interviews, with similar findings. It was found that models containing carbon monoxide, rather than tar or nicotine, tended to explain the greatest amount of variability. Consumption at 28 weeks was more closely related to reduction in ABWR than that at booking or 36 weeks.

Several other modelling approaches were tried. In one of these the number of cigarettes was multiplied by the yield to obtain a measure of total exposure to the constituent. Linear regression of ABWR on this variable obtained a flat gradient that, when extrapolated to non-smokers, predicted less effect on ABWR than observed in reality. This was improved by using a quadratic or

**Table 8.3** Mean adjusted birth weight ratio by alcohol and caffeine consumption in all women, and by smoking status at booking

| Factor | All women | | Non-smokers | | Smokers | | Significance of $F$ ratio | |
|---|---|---|---|---|---|---|---|---|
| | Number* | ABWR | Number* | ABWR | Number* | ABWR | | |
| Alcohol (g/week) | | | | | | | | |
| 0 | 759 | 1.042 | 548 | 1.050 | 211 | 1.020 | All women: linear trend | $P = 0.04$ |
| 1–19 | 381 | 1.037 | 258 | 1.052 | 123 | 1.007 | Alcohol adj for smoking | $P = 0.74$ |
| 20–49 | 249 | 1.032 | 148 | 1.061 | 101 | 0.990 | Smoking adj for alcohol | $P < 0.001$ |
| 50–99 | 81 | 1.023 | 50 | 1.056 | 31 | 0.970 | Linear trend non-smokers | $P = 0.31$ |
| 100+ | 40 | 1.003 | 16 | 1.082 | 24 | 0.951 | Linear trend smokers | $P = 0.003$ |
| Tea (cups/week) | | | | | | | | |
| 0 | 210 | 1.050 | 144 | 1.059 | 67 | 1.030 | All women; linear trend | $P = 0.004$ |
| 1–14 | 512 | 1.043 | 392 | 1.052 | 120 | 1.013 | Tea adj smoking, | $P = 0.32$ |
| | | | | | | | Smoking adj tea | $P < 0.001$ |
| 15–42 | 645 | 1.034 | 429 | 1.053 | 216 | 0.997 | Linear trend non-smokers | $P = 0.52$ |
| | | | | | | | Linear trend smokers | $P < 0.04$ |

|  | 140 | 1.012 | 53 | 1.046 | 87 | 0.992 |  |  |
| 43+ |  |  |  |  |  |  |  |  |
| Coffee (cups/week) |  |  |  |  |  |  |  |  |
| 0 | 506 | 1.038 | 360 | 1.050 | 146 | 1.008 | All women; linear trend | $P = 0.003$ |
| 1–7 | 549 | 1.041 | 394 | 1.050 | 155 | 1.017 | Coffee adj smoking | $P = 0.12$ |
|  |  |  |  |  |  |  | Smoking adj coffee | $P < 0.001$ |
| 8–28 | 343 | 1.042 | 221 | 1.065 | 122 | 1.00 | Linear trend non-smokers | $P = 0.51$ |
| 29+ | 112 | 0.997 | 44 | 1.032 | 68 | 0.975 | Linear trend smokers | $P = 0.04$ |
| Total caffeine (mg/week) |  |  |  |  |  |  |  |  |
| 0–1400 | 405 | 1.050 | 335 | 1.052 | 70 | 1.043 | All women; linear trend | $P = 0.001$ |
|  |  |  |  |  |  |  | Caffeine adj smoking | $P = 0.26$ |
|  |  |  |  |  |  |  | Smoking adj caffeine | $P < 0.001$ |
| 1401–2800 | 591 | 1.041 | 420 | 1.051 | 171 | 1.016 | Linear trend non-smokers | $P = 0.57$ |
| $\geq 2801$ | 509 | 1.023 | 261 | 1.058 | 248 | 0.986 | Linear trend smokers | $P < 0.001$ |

* Reduced number of subjects due to missing histories.
ABWR, adjusted birth weight ratio.

**Table 8.4** Fitting linear models of adjusted birth weight on cigarettes smoked and their constituents at 28 weeks among consistent smokers ($n = 340$)

| Model: independent variables | Regression coefficient[1] | 95% CI | $t$-test | Equivalent change in BW[2] | $R^2$ |
|---|---|---|---|---|---|
| 1. Cigs/day | −0.190 | −0.36, −0.027 | $p = 0.02$ | −7 | 0.015 |
| 2. CO | −0.480 | −0.85, −0.120 | $P = 0.01$ | −17 | 0.020 |
| 3. Cigs/day | −0.170 | −0.33, 0.001 | $P = 0.05$ | −6 | 0.031 |
|    CO | −0.430 | −0.80, −0.069 | $P = 0.02$ | −15 | |
| 4. Cigs/day | −0.610 | −1.48, 0.260 | $P = 0.20$ | −21 | 0.034 |
|    CO | −0.710 | −1.36, −0.060 | $P = 0.03$ | −25 | |
|    Cigs*CO | 0.028 | −0.026, 0.081 | $P = 0.30$ | 1 | |
| 5. Tar | −0.470 | −0.10, −0.850 | $P = 0.01$ | −17 | 0.018 |
| 6. Cigs/day | −0.170 | −0.34, −0.003 | $P = 0.05$ | −6 | 0.029 |
|    Tar | −0.430 | −0.80, −0.049 | $P = 0.03$ | −15 | |
| 7. Cigs/day | −0.570 | −1.44, 0.300 | $P = 0.20$ | −20 | 0.032 |
|    Tar | −0.680 | −1.36, −0.010 | $P = 0.05$ | −24 | |
|    Cigs*tar | 0.026 | −0.030, 0.081 | $P = 0.40$ | 1 | |
| 8. Nicotine | −6.210 | −11.34, −1.08 | $P = 0.02$ | −217 | 0.016 |
| 9. Cigs/day | −0.170 | −0.34, 0.002 | $P = 0.05$ | −6 | 0.028 |
|    Nicotine | −5.490 | −10.65, −0.330 | $P = 0.04$ | −192 | |
| 10. Cigs/day | −0.850 | −1.90, 0.200 | $P = 0.10$ | −30 | 0.032 |
|    Nicotine | −10.510 | −19.74, −1.270 | $P = 0.03$ | −367 | |
|    Cigs*nic | 0.520 | −0.27, 1.300 | $P = 0.20$ | 18 | |

[1] Regression coefficient is % change in birth weight per unit.
Units for carbon monoxide (CO), tar, nicotine are mg/cig.
[2] Equivalent change in birth weight is in g at term (40 weeks).

logarithmic transform but at this stage a different approach was tried and, in the event, gave as good a fit as these latter techniques.

Plots of the number of cigarettes against each of the constituents revealed a triangular pattern from which three main and one minor groups of smokers could be discerned:

(1) low number of cigarettes and low yield;
(2) low number of cigarettes and high yield;
(3) high number of cigarettes and low yield;
(4) high number of cigarettes and high yield.

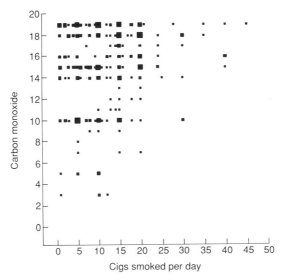

Fig. 8.1. Scatter diagram of carbon monoxide yield by number of cigarettes smoked at 28 weeks gestation.

This is shown in Fig. 8.1 for carbon monoxide at 28 weeks. From looking at the plots, an arbitrary cut off of 15 cigarettes per day was chosen to divide high and low numbers of cigarettes. From among the constituents, carbon monoxide was chosen with a cut-off point of $< 12$ mg defining low yield and 12 mg or more defining high yield. The cut-off point for carbon monoxide corresponded fairly closely to the upper boundary for 'low tar' cigarettes. Analysis of ABWR using these categories is shown in Table 8.5 for each interview. It is seen that the ABWRs of the low cigarettes/low yield group were similar to those of non-smokers. In contrast, the other three groups had similar low values of ABWR. As was found in the previous linear regression analysis, the greatest amount of variation in ABWR was explained by the 28-week data and the least by the 36-week data.

Analysis was done after further subdividing the women according to consistency across the three interviews in brand and in numbers of cigarettes smoked (Table 8.6). It was found that non-smokers and consistent smokers of less than 15 cigarettes per day of a low-yield brand had similar mean ABWRs of about 1.055. Women who smoked throughout pregnancy, who did not change smoking group, and who smoked 15+ cigarettes day, or who smoked a high-yield brand or both all had a mean birth weight between 4 and 9 per cent lower. The lowest mean ABWR was for the group of women whose smoking habit varied but was always above the low cigarettes/low yield cut-off. Inconsistent smoking was associated with little reduction in ABWR. Those who never reported smoking either low number of cigarettes or low

**Table 8.5** Mean adjusted birth weight by smoking group for booking, 28, and 36 weeks amongst those with consistent smoking habits*

| Smoking group | Booking | | 28 weeks | | 36 weeks | |
|---|---|---|---|---|---|---|
| | Number | Mean | Number | Mean | Number | Mean |
| Low cigs Low yield | 51 | 1.052 | 53 | 1.056 | 59 | 1.036 |
| Low cigs High yield | 179 | 0.995 | 152 | 0.994 | 153 | 0.997 |
| High cigs Low yield | 14 | 0.960 | 19 | 0.978 | 23 | 0.964 |
| High cigs High yield | 96 | 0.986 | 116 | 0.985 | 105 | 0.991 |
| Non-smokers | 895 | 1.050 | 895 | 1.050 | 895 | 1.050 |

* Reported smoking at each interview or non-smoking at each interview.

yield had the lowest ABWR (0.958). We concluded from this analysis that a threshold existed whereby women smoking below this level had a similar mean ABWR to non-smokers.

Further analysis was carried out to determine the exact threshold values using maximum likelihood methods (Peacock 1989) and a threshold value of 13 cigarettes per day and 15 mg carbon monoxide were obtained. For those below the threshold the mean ABWR was 1.063, for those above the threshold the mean ABWR was 0.984, a difference of 8 per cent or 280 g at term.

Trends in ABWR with numbers of cigarettes and with each of the three constituents were examined within women smoking below and above the threshold, respectively, and none were significant, thus further supporting the existence of a threshold.

Previous analyses using linear regression had found that within smokers the effects of alcohol and caffeine persisted after controlling for the number of cigarettes smoked. Because the threshold model fitted the data better than a linear one, the effects of these factors were re-examined within smokers using the threshold for quantity and brand as described above to control for smoking. Using multiple regression analysis, the independent effect of each factor—smoking, alcohol, and caffeine—was examined for each of the three interviews (Table 8.7). At booking, all three factors were significant after controlling for the others. Heavy smokers (high numbers of cigarettes or high yield) had a reduction of 5 per cent in birth weight compared with light

**Table 8.6** Mean adjusted birth weight by eight smoking groups*

| Smoking groups | Number | Mean | 95%   CI |
|---|---|---|---|
| Non-smokers | 895 | 1.050 | 1.042, 1.058 |
| Low cigs/low yield throughout | 36 | 1.062 | 1.021, 1.103 |
| Low cigs/high yield throughout | 109 | 0.999 | 0.976, 1.023 |
| High cigs/low yield throughout | 10 | 0.975 | 0.897, 1.052 |
| High cigs/high yield throughout | 64 | 1.009 | 0.979, 1.040 |
| Inconsistent smokers | 74 | 1.038 | 1.010, 1.066 |
| Change groups including low cigs/low yield at some time | 42 | 1.015 | 0.977, 1.052 |
| Change groups between low cigs/low yield, high cigs/low yield, and high cigs/high yield, i.e. never low cigs/low yield | 79 | 0.958 | 0.931, 0.986 |

* $< 15/15+$ cigs per day, $< 12\,mg/12\,mg + CO$ per cigarette.

smokers after controlling for the other factors. The heaviest drinkers had reductions of 8 per cent compared with non-drinkers and women consuming $> 2800\,mg$/week of caffeine had a reduction of 4 per cent. At 28 weeks the effects of smoking and caffeine remained but that of alcohol (3 per cent for all drinkers) was less and showed no trend. At 36 weeks, the effect of smoking was less and those of alcohol and caffeine were non-significant, though still negative.

## Discussion

The findings of this study may be summarized as follows:

1. Smoking in pregnancy was associated with reduced fetal growth.
2. The association between smoking and fetal growth was best described by a threshold model than by linear or logarithmic models.
3. The yield of cigarette was more closely related to reduction in fetal growth than numbers of cigarettes.

**Table 8.7** Multiple regression analysis of effects of smoking, alcohol, and caffeine consumption on mean adjusted birth weight ratio

| | Booking (n = 471) | | 28 weeks (n = 431) | | 36 weeks (n = 413) | |
|---|---|---|---|---|---|---|
| | Adjusted mean difference in ABWR | P value | Adjusted mean difference in ABWR | P value | Adjusted mean difference in ABWR | P value |
| Smoking* | | | | | | |
| Heavy smoker | −0.051 | P < 0.001 | −0.050 | P < 0.001 | −0.034 | P = 0.02 |
| Alcohol† (g/week) | | | | | | |
| 1–19 | −0.016 | | −0.045 | | −0.021 | |
| 20–49 | −0.035 | | −0.030 | | −0.034 | |
| 50–99 | −0.047 | P < 0.01 | −0.005 | P = 0.07 | −0.030 | P = 0.24 |
| 100+ | −0.081 | | −0.028 | | −0.024 | |
| Caffeine‡ (mg/week) | | | | | | |
| 1401–2800 | −0.016 | | −0.060 | | −0.023 | |
| 2801+ | −0.044 | P = 0.01 | −0.065 | P < 0.01 | −0.039 | P = 0.10 |

* Compared with light smokers (< 13 cigs/day and < 15 mg/cig carbon monoxide).
† Compared with non-drinkers.
‡ Compared with intake ≤ 1400 mg/week.
ABWR adjusted birth weight ratio.

4. An effect of alcohol on fetal growth was observed but only in smokers.
5. An effect of caffeine on fetal growth was observed but only in smokers.
6. Within smokers the relationships with alcohol and caffeine persisted when smoking was controlled using the model incorporating both numbers of cigarettes and yield of brand smoked.
7. Of the large number of psychosocial factors examined, very few were associated with reduced fetal growth and all these were explained by smoking.

Overall, the existence and size of the smoking effect observed in this study resembled that in many other studies (US Department of Health and Human Services 1980). What is more interesting is the nature of the relationship with the number of cigarettes smoked and brand. Where this has been examined by previous workers a plateau or logarithmic relationship has usually been reported (Andrews and McGarry 1972; Kline *et al.* 1987). In many studies the relationship has not been examined and for the purposes of analysis has been assumed to be linear. The authors are not aware of any other studies that have attempted to analyse the effects of quantity and yield together. It is concluded that, in this population, the yield of the cigarette, as defined by the Government Chemist, must be taken into consideration if the observed data are to be adequately explained. Women smoking low numbers of low-yield cigarettes had babies of similar size to those of non-smokers, while those who smoked low numbers of high-yield cigarettes had babies whose growth had been retarded to the same extent as those who smoked higher quantities.

It must be emphasized that the existence of the threshold and the value of the cut-off point were both derived empirically, not hypothesized a priori; for this reason, the findings must not be generalized to other populations. They do, however, provide a hypothesis that requires testing in new studies. These will require greater statistical power and it would be highly desirable to incorporate objective methods of measuring intake of tobacco smoke, such as urinary cotinine or blood carboxyhaemoglobin estimations. It would also be highly desirable to measure other outcomes, such as congenital defects and abnormalities of early development.

The effects of nicotine and carbon monoxide have been studied extensively in pregnant women and animal experiments and there is little doubt that both are potential causes of impaired fetal growth. Nicotine reduces uteroplacental blood flow, increases catecholamine levels, and may reduce uptake of nutrients by the placenta; it passes rapidly into the fetal circulation. Smoking results in levels of carboxyhaemoglobin of up to 10 per cent and it has been estimated that at this level the fetus is exposed to serious reductions in oxygen transport (Longo 1977). Of course, there are many other potential toxins, including hydrogen cyanide, polycyclic aromatic hydrocarbons, oxides of nitrogen, and cadmium, but little is known about their role in reducing fetal growth.

The existence of a threshold effect is biologically plausible. It could, for example, result from a failure of homeostatic mechanisms to compensate for toxicological stress after a critical level is reached. Longo (1977), in reviewing the effects of carbon monoxide, has pointed out that there may be a critical point at which reduced capillary oxygen tension begins to cause hypoxic effects. In studies of the aerobic metabolism of exercising skeletal muscle, there is a threshold of 5 per cent carboxyhaemoglobin above which tissue hypoxia begins to occur.

Attempts were made to examine the relative importance of the three constituents described by the Government Chemist for each brand. However, because of the strong intercorrelation between nicotine, tar, and carbon monoxide the study could yield little useful information about which of the constituents might be more important. It was noted, however, that linear models at 28 weeks that included carbon monoxide explained more of the variability in ABWR than any of those which included nicotine or tar.

Other investigations of the effects of alcohol on birth weight that have controlled for smoking have found no effect (Beaulac-Baillargeon and Desrosiers 1987; Sulaiman *et al.* 1988), a slight effect (Kline *et al.* 1987) or an effect (Kaminski *et al.* 1978; Mills *et al.* 1984; Fried and O'Connell 1987). One study, carried out in a neighbouring borough to Wandsworth found a similar effect of alcohol in smokers only (Wright *et al.* 1983). Thus there is evidence of an interaction between smoking and alcohol consumption. This finding is in line with some studies of other outcomes in pregnancy (Martin *et al.* 1977) and some animal experiments (Leichter 1989) and has been attributed partly to reduced food intake. Unlike animal studies, there was no effect of alcohol in the absence of smoking. The effect was strongest at booking.

Also found was an effect of caffeine consumption on fetal growth. This was independent of the association of caffeine with alcohol and smoking use and is in line with the findings of Mau and Netter (1974), Watkinson and Fried (1985), Beaulac-Baillargeon and Desrosiers (1987), and Martin and Bracken (1987), but not with those of Van den Berg (1977) and Fried and O'Connell (1987). Thus, in smokers, the effects of alcohol and caffeine are additive such that if, when booking, a woman is smoking over the threshold of either yield (15+ mg carbon monoxide per cigarette) or number of cigarettes (13+ cigarettes per day), and is a heavy drinker (100+ g/week)—just under two drinks per day—and has a high caffeine intake (2801+ mg/week), her predicted reduction in birth weight would be 18 per cent.

The St George's Birthweight study was very comprehensive, and careful attention was paid to the quality of data collection, measurement of possibly confounding variables, correction of birthweight for gestational age, and modelling of the smoking relationship. Its findings, if generally applicable, would have considerable public health importance and implications for health education. They must be tested using further studies in which there is sufficient statistical power to look at these factors in more detail, at other outcomes and using objective measures of smoke exposure.

# Acknowledgements

We wish to thank Professors R R Trussell and G V P Chamberlain, the clinic staff for facilitating this study, and all the interviewers and participants. We also wish to thank Dr O G Brooke, who was responsible for initiating the research, and Mr M Stewart who, as research fellow, organized the data collection. Financial support was received from a consortium of American Tobacco Companies.

# References

Abel, E. L. (1980). Smoking during pregnancy: A review of effects on growth and development of offspring. *Human Biology*, **52**, 593–625.

Al-Samarrae, W., Ma, M. C. F., and Truswell, A. S. (1975). Methylxanthine consumption from coffee and tea. *Proceedings of the Nutrition Society*, **34**, 18A–19A.

Andrews, J. and McGarry, J. M. (1972). A community study of smoking in pregnancy. *Journal of Obstetrics and Gynaecology of the British Commonwealth*, **79**, 1057–73.

Beaulac-Baillargeon, L. and Desrosiers, C. (1987). Caffeine cigarette interaction on fetal growth. *American Journal of Obstetrics and Gynaecology*, **157**, 1236–40.

Bland, J. M., Peacock, J. L., Anderson, H. R., Brooke, O. G., and DeCurtis, M. (1990). The adjustment of birthweight for very early gestational ages. *Applied Statistics*, **39**, 229–39.

Brooke, O. G., Anderson, H. R., Bland, J. M., Peacock, J. L., and Stewart, C. M. (1989). Effects on birth weight of smoking, alcohol, caffeine, socioeconomic factors, and psychosocial stress. *British Medical Journal*, **298**, 795–801.

Butler, N. R., Goldstein, H., and Ross, E. M. (1972). Cigarette smoking in pregnancy: its influence on birth weight and perinatal mortality. *British Medical Journal*, **ii**, 127–30.

Dunn, H. G. (1984). Social aspects of low birthweight. *Canadian Medical Association Journal*, **130**, 1131–40.

Fried, P. A. and O'Connell, C. M. (1987). A comparison of the effects of prenatal exposure to tobacco, alcohol, cannabis and caffeine on birth size and subsequent growth. *Neurotoxicology and Teratology*, **9**, 79–85.

Goldberg, D. P. and Hillier, V. F. (1979). A scale version of the general health questionnaire. *Psychological Medicine*, **9**, 139–45.

Graham, D. M. (1978). Caffeine—its identity, dietary sources, intake and biological effects. *Nutrition Reviews*, **36**, 97–102.

Heller, J., Anderson, H. R., Bland, J. M., Brooke, O. G., Peacock, J. L., and Stewart, C. M. (1988). Alcohol in pregnancy: patterns and association with socioeconomic, psychological and behavioural factors. *British Journal of Addiction*, **83**, 541–51.

Kaminski, M., Rumeau, C., and Schwartz, D. (1978). Alcohol consumption in pregnant women and the outcome of pregnancy. *Alcoholism: Clinical and Experimental Research*, **2**, 155–63.

Keen, D. V. and Pearse, R. G. (1985). Birthweight between 14 and 42 weeks' gestation. *Archives of Disease in Childhood*, **60**, 440–6.

Kline, J., Stein, K., and Hutzler, M. (1987). Cigarettes, alcohol and Marijuana. Varying associations with birthweight. *International Journal of Epidemiology*, **16**, 44–51.

Leichter, J. (1989). Growth of fetuses of rats exposed to ethanol and cigarette smoke during gestation. *Growth, Development and Aging*, **53**, 129–34.

Longo, L. D. (1977). The biological effects of carbon monoxide on the pregnant woman, fetus, and newborn infant. *American Journal of Obstetrics and Gynecology*, **129**, 69–103.

MacArthur, C. and Knox, E. G. (1988). Smoking in pregnancy: effects of stopping at different stages. *British Journal of Obstetrics and Gynaecology*, **95**, 551–5.

Martin, T. R. and Bracken, M. B. (1987). The association between low birthweight and caffeine consumption during pregnancy. *American Journal of Epidemiology*, **126**, 813–21.

Martin, J., Martin, D. C., Lund, C. A., and Streissguth, A. P. (1977). Maternal alcohol ingestion and cigarette smoking and their effects on newborn conditioning. *Alcoholism*, **1**, 243–7.

Mau, G. and Netter, P. (1974). Are coffee and alcohol consumption risk factors in pregnancy? *Geburtsch u Frauenheilk*, **34**, 1018–22.

McIntosh, I. D. (1984). Smoking and pregnancy: II. Offspring risks. *Public Health Reviews*, **12**, 29–63.

Mills, J. L., Graubard, B. I., Harley, E. E., Rhoads, G. G., and Berendes, H. W. (1984). Maternal alcohol consumption and birthweight. How much drinking during pregnancy is safe? *Journal of the American Medical Association*, **252**, 1875–9.

Oster, G., Delea, T. E., and Colditz, G. A. (1988). Maternal smoking during pregnancy and expenditures on neonatal health care. *American Journal of Preventive Medicine*, **4**, 216–19.

Paul, A. A. and Southgate, D. A. T. (1978). *McCance and Widdowson's the composition of foods*, (4th edn). HMSO, London.

Paykel, E. S., Myers, K. J., Dienelt, M. N., Lerman, G. L., Lindenthal, J. J., and Pepper, M. P. (1969). Life events and depression: a controlled study. *Archives of General Psychiatry*, **21**, 753–60.

Peacock, J. L. (1989). *Birthweight and cigarette smoking*. PhD thesis, University of London.

Peacock, J. L., Bland, J. M., and Anderson, H. R. (1991). Effects on birthweight of alcohol and caffeine consumption in smoking women. *Journal of Epidemiology and Community Health*, **45**, 159–63.

Picone, T. A., Allen, L. H., Olsen, P. N., and Ferris, M. E. (1982). Pregnancy outcome in North American women. 2. Effects of diet, cigarette smoking, stress and weight gain on placentas, and on neonatal physical and behavioural characteristics. *American Journal of Clinical Nutrition*, **36**, 1214–24.

Rush, D. and Cassano, P. (1983). Relationship between cigarette smoking and social class to birthweight and perinatal mortality among all births in Britain, 5–11 April 1970. *Journal of Epidemiology and Community Health*, **37**, 249–55.

Simpson, W. J. (1957). A preliminary report on cigarette smoking and the incidence of prematurity. *American Journal of Obstetrics and Gynecology*, **73**, 808–15.

Sulaiman, N. D., Florey, C. du V., Taylor, D. J., and Ogston, S. A. (1988). Alcohol consumption in Dundee primigravidas and its effect on outcome of pregnancy. *British Medical Journal*, **296**, 1500–3.

UK Department of Health (1983). *Tar, carbon monoxide and nicotine yields of cigarettes*. HMSO, London.

US Department of Health and Human Services (1980). *The health consequences of smoking for women: a report of the Surgeon General*. US Department of Health and Human Services, Office on Smoking and Health, Rockville, Maryland.

US Department of Health and Human Services (1981). *The health consequences of smoking—the changing cigarette. A report of the Surgeon General.* US Department of Health and Human Services, Rockville, Maryland.

Van den Berg, B. J. (1977). Epidemiological observations of prematurity: effects of tobacco, coffee and alcohol. In *Epidemiology of prematurity*, (ed. D. M. Reed and R. J. Stanley), pp. 157–76. Urban and Schwartzenberg, Baltimore.

Watkinson, B. and Fried, P. A. (1985). Maternal caffeine use before, during and after pregnancy and effects upon offspring. *Neurobehavioural Toxicology and Teratology,* **7,** 9–17.

Wright, J. T., Waterson, E. J., and Barrison, I. G. (1983). Alcohol consumption, pregnancy and low birthweight. *Lancet,* **i,** 663–5.

Yerushalmy, J. (1971). The relationship of parents' cigarette smoking to outcome of pregnancy—implications as to the problem of inferring causation from observed associations. *American Journal of Epidemiology,* **93,** 443–56.

# 9. A preliminary analysis of interactions between smoking and infant feeding

*Jonathan I Pollock*

## Introduction

Although many reports exist in the epidemiological literature linking maternal smoking to unfavourable, and breast-feeding to favourable outcomes in the child, the strong negative associations these two types of maternal behaviour have with each other and with psychosocial and socio-economic circumstances have rarely been allowed for. However, given a sufficient sample size and a broad database, multivariate techniques enable researchers to separate more efficiently individual influences from confounding factors, and to examine statistical interactions between them. It is possible, therefore, not only to look at associations between smoking or breast-feeding and child health and development in a more rigorously controlled fashion, but also to test the hypothesis that the effects of maternal smoking may be different in infants fed in different ways. This is of topical interest because although the rates of smoking in women of childbearing age have levelled out recently (Office of Population Censuses and Surveys 1988), breast-feeding in the United Kingdom (Martin and White 1988) and in much of the Western world has risen substantially from its lowest prevalence, reached in the early 1970s. Although smokers are less likely to breast-feed their babies than non-smokers a large population of mothers exists who both smoke and breast-feed.

The purpose of this chapter is to examine interations between maternal smoking and infant feeding by presenting evidence relevant to two central questions:

1. Is maternal smoking itself independently associated with breast- or bottle-feeding.
2. Are the associations between maternal smoking and child health and development different in breast-fed and bottle-fed children.

## Does maternal smoking have a direct influence on breast-feeding?

### Published reports

In Western populations breast-feeding and smoking are both predicted by the same social factors, albeit in different directions, and it is to be expected that strong relationships exist between them. Higher initial and long-term breast-feeding rates were found in non-smokers by Whichelow and King (1979), Yeung *et al.* (1981), and Lyon (1983). In each case breast-feeding differentials between smokers and non-smokers increased with infant age, indicating that not only did fewer smoking mothers start breast-feeding but they ceased breast-feeding earlier. Dose–response relationships between smoking rates and breast-feeding were evident in the studies by Lyon (1983) and Woodward and Hand (1988) and the associations determined by Whichelow and King (1979) and Lyon (1983) remained after adjusting for social class. A recent study in Norway, conducted by Nylander and Matheson (1989), also showed a dose–response relationship between smoking and the prevalence of breast-feeding and indicated that more smokers than non-smokers reported having stopped breast-feeding because of having 'too little milk'. This study, however, made no attempt to adjust for confounding factors.

These data are all consistent with the hypothesis that both initial breast-feeding and continued breast-feeding may be directly influenced by maternal smoking behaviour. However, only one study has attempted to control for confounding factors with any degree of rigour. This study by Woodward and Hand (1988) adjusted not only for social class but also for low birth weight and reported illness in the infant, all of which may be important factors influencing a mother's choice or ability to breast-feed.

## Analysis of the British Births Survey

*Initial breast-feeding*   A recent analysis of the 1970 British Births Survey, a longitudinal study of one week's births throughout the United Kingdom (Chamberlain *et al.* 1975), included a multivariate examination of factors associated with both smoking and breast-feeding. The first step in this analysis was to ascertain if the mother's smoking habit explained some of the residual variance in breast-feeding once other independent predictors had been held constant. Twins were excluded and mothers of first and subequent births looked at separately, as breast-feeding was expected to have different predictors in first-time mothers than in those with experience of parenting. The criterion used for initial breast-feeding was 'any breast-feeding during the infant's first week', and the criterion for smoking was 'smoking at any time in pregnancy'. Although the smoking groups in this analysis related to maternal smoking during pregnancy, the vast majority (93.8 per cent) continued smoking in the postnatal period.

A total of 62 background factors relating to the social, economic, regional, and biological characteristics of the mother, her partner, and their families, and the mother's reproductive and clinical history were used in the analysis. Groups of these background variables were subjected to a series of stepwise logistic regression equations to select a model of best-fitting independent predictors. The mother's smoking habits were included in the modelling procedure and in both parity groups this factor remained as a significant ($P < 0.01$) independent predictor.

The odds of the mother starting to breast-feed in those who stopped smoking before or during pregnancy and those who smoked throughout pregnancy (compared to non-smokers) are presented in Table 9.1. For both parity groups women who stopped smoking before, or at some time during, pregnancy had a slightly higher rate of initial breast-feeding than non-smokers, but smokers had significantly lower rates.

It is probable that women who stopped smoking during pregnancy or even before pregnancy are more motivated to engage in other forms of positive health behaviour, a relationship that may be responsible for their increased initial breast-feeding rates.

**Table 9.1** Odds of any breast feeding in first week in smokers and non-smokers adjusted for other factors

| | Adjusted odds ratio and 99% confidence limits | $\chi^2(2df)^*$ | $P$ |
|---|---|---|---|
| Primiparae ($n = 5917$)† | | | |
| Non-smoker[a] | 1 | 15.49 | 0.0004 |
| Stopped before/ during pregnancy | 1.17 (1.03, 1.33) | | |
| Smoked throughout pregnancy | 0.85 (0.76, 0.95) | | |
| Multiparae ($n = 9864$)‡ | | | |
| Non-smoker[a] | 1 | 21.27 | < 0.0001 |
| Stopped before/ during pregnancy | 1.11 (0.99, 1.25) | | |
| Smoked throughout pregnancy | 0.84 (0.76, 0.93) | | |

* $\chi^2$ refers to heterogeneity of the whole group
† Adjusted for: Region of birth, maternal social class, maternal education, maternal height, mother's region of birth, contraceptive use, pre-marital conception, antenatal parentcraft class attendance, and incubation of infant
‡ Adjusted for: Region of birth, maternal and paternal social class, paternal education, maternal age, mother's region of birth, contraceptive use, antenatal labour preparation class attendance, and incubation of infant
a = Reference group

*Continued breast-feeding* Amongst the women who started breast-feeding it is pertinent to ask whether the duration of lactation/breast-feeding is also related to their smoking behaviour. A similar modelling procedure was conducted in the same two parity groups. The criterion for long-term breast-feeding was 'breast-feeding, wholly or partially, which continued for longer than 1 month'.

The results (Table 9.2) indicate a discrepancy between parity groups in their relationship between smoking and continued breast-feeding. For the 2201 primiparous women who started breast-feeding no significant association with smoking could be determined after adjusting for the five independent predictors of prolonged breast-feeding. For the 2531 multiparous women a significantly reduced incidence of long-term breast-feeding was found in the group who had smoked at any time during pregnancy, after adjusting for the six other independent predictors (Table 9.2). Other studies of this cohort have shown that there were more heavy smokers in the multiparous than primiparous group (Evans 1989). It is possible, therefore, that the parity difference in this result is related to different dose exposures.

The results of these analyses indicate that maternal smoking appears to have significant predictive value in initial and, for multiparae, long-term breast-feeding, once other factors associated with each form of infant feeding are held constant.

It remains uncertain, however, whether it is smoking itself or some factor closely linked to smoking that is responsible for its association with breast-feeding. This latter contingency was explored by creating a model, for each parity group, of factors independently predictive of maternal smoking in preg-

**Table 9.2** Odds of breast-feeding for longer than 1 month in smokers and non-smokers adjusted for other factors

|  | Adjusted odds ratio and 99% confidence limits | $\chi^2(2df)^*$ | *P* |
|---|---|---|---|
| Primiparae ($n = 2201$)[†] |  |  |  |
| Non-smoker[‡] | 1 | 0.02 | 0.9912 |
| Stopped before/ during pregnancy | 1.01 (0.82, 1.24) |  |  |
| Smoker | 1.00 (0.82, 1.21) |  |  |
| Multiparae ($n = 2531$)[§] |  |  |  |
| Non-smoker[a] | 1 | 12.74 | 0.0017 |
| Stopped before/ during pregnancy | 1.12 (0.92, 1.35) |  |  |
| Smoker | 0.80 (0.68, 0.94) |  |  |

\* $\chi^2$ refers to heterogeneity of the whole group.
† Adjusted for: Region of birth, maternal social class, maternal age, maternal education, antenatal labour preparation class attendance.
§ Adjusted for: Region of birth, paternal social class, father's place of birth, maternal education, inpatient admissions in pregnancy, birthweight of index child.
‡ Reference group.

nancy and, holding these constant, computing the odds of breast-feeding in the mothers who had smoked. Once adjusted for other independent predictors of maternal smoking the chances of being breast-fed initially, and being breast-fed for longer than 1 month were both substantially and significantly lower in the group whose mothers smoked during pregnancy, with the possible exception of long-term breast-feeding in the primiparous group (Table 9.3).

These results are consistent with an independent effect of smoking on lactation and/or breast-feeding. This raises the question of whether the putative mechanism is direct or indirect. As reported from animal (rat) studies (Ferry *et al.* 1974), basal levels of serum prolactin in pregnancy are lower in women smoking cigarettes than in non-smokers (Andersen *et al.* 1982), although these authors found that nursing the infant induced increments in serum prolactin that were independent of smoking status. Later work by this group indicated that the lower basal prolactin levels in pregnancy in cigarette smokers could be due to either a direct effect of nicotine or to a secondary effect of reduced levels of oestrogen (Andersen *et al.* 1984). The suggestion of a direct effect of smoking on oxytocin release via an inhibitory action of adrenalin (Cross 1955) was not supported by the work of Andersen *et al.*

**Table 9.3** Odds of being breast-fed in the group whose mothers smoked at all during pregnancy adjusted for factors predictive of smoking

|  | Primiparae* | Multiparae† |
|---|---|---|
| Breast-fed in the first week | | |
|    Adjusted odds ratio | 0.84 | 0.77 |
|    95% confidence limits | 0.75, 0.95 | 0.70, 0.85 |
|    $\chi^2(1\mathrm{df})$ | 7.72 | 26.09 |
|    $P$ | 0.0055 | <0.0001 |
| Breast-fed for > 1 month in those mothers who started breast-feeding | | |
|    Adjusted odds ratio | 0.85 | 0.68 |
|    95% confidence limits | 0.72, 1.00 | 0.59, 0.77 |
|    $\chi^2(1\mathrm{df})$ | 4.08 | 32.38 |
|    $P$ | 0.0434 | <0.0001 |

* Factors adjusted for: region of birth, mother's place of birth, mother's social class, education, father's employment status, marital status at conception.
† Factors adjusted for: region of delivery, mother's place of birth, mother's social class, education, age, father's occupational class, contraception used, number of previous pregnancies, inter-birth interval.

(1982). A further possible direct mechanism may be through the inhibition of lipogenesis by nicotine reducing the production of breast milk (Topping 1980). Indirect effects may also play a role through, for example disturbances of the mother–infant relationship. The sucking response that stimulates lacto-genesis may be reduced in the infants of mothers who smoked during preg-nancy (Martin *et al.* 1979), which may limit the duration of breast-feeding. More 'colic and excessive crying' in the 3-month-old infants of breast-feeding smokers compared with those of breast-feeding non-smokers has been recently reported (Nylander and Matheson 1989) and this may affect decisions to continue breast-feeding.

In conclusion, the relatively small amount of epidemiological data available indicates that at least part of the association between smoking behaviour on the one hand and lower rates and reduced duration of breast-feeding on the other may be a result of an interference with the process of lactation and/or breast-feeding. Should a direct physiological suppression be involved a focused research project would be needed to identify possible mechanisms.

## Are there any interactions between maternal smoking and type of infant feeding in relation to the outcome of pregnancy and long-term associations in the child?

This question is concerned with testing the hypothesis that mothers who breast-feed their child and smoke are putting their infant at risk to a different degree to those who smoke and bottle-feed. An examination of the literature on smoking and child outcomes failed to identify any studies that directly addressed this question. Consequently, an analysis was conducted using data from the British Births Survey and subsequent Child Health and Education Study of the cohort at 5 and 10 years of age (see Butler and Golding 1986), to seek long-term associations with smoking in breast-feeding and bottle-feeding mothers.

The methods employed are similar to those presented in the first part of this chapter. Separate best-fitting models were created by stepwise logistic re-gression analysis for identifying independent factors associated with maternal smoking in pregnancy in those women who subsequently breast-fed their children for at least 1 month and those who bottle-fed their baby from birth. Social, biological, and behavioural characteristics of the mother and events in pregnancy and delivery were related to the mother's smoking behaviour and needed to be adjusted for.

Certain differences between the breast-feeding and bottle-feeding groups, however, were expected to interfere with direct comparisons of the results. First, the proportion of women who smoked throughout the pregnancy of the index child, and the number of cigarettes smoked each day, differed in the two infant feeding groups. Subsequent breast-feeders were more likely to have given up smoking during pregnancy and to have smoked fewer cigarettes per day (Table 9.4). Because of the confounding issue of postnatal smoking, even in those who did not smoke in pregnancy, the examination of associations reported at 5 and 10 years of age was restricted to mothers who did not smoke in pregnancy or up to the time the index child was 5 years of age, and mothers who smoked both during pregnancy and up to their child's fifth birthday. This reduced the sample size, but the relative differences in the percentage who gave up during pregnancy and in the dosage of cigarette smoking between breast-feeders and bottle-feeders remained similar (Table 9.4). The present analysis is therefore unable to compare for breast- and bottle-feeding groups the effects of dose or time of smoking during pregnancy. Examination of dose–response relationships in comparing the effects of maternal smoking in breast-feeding and bottle-feeding groups is currently underway.

## Associations in pregnancy or at birth

Of the 39 associations examined between maternal smoking and events during pregnancy or delivery only five were found to be significant ($P < 0.01$) in one or other feeding group (Table 9.5). For both breast-feeding and bottle-feeding groups maternal smoking was associated to approximately the same degree with an increase in the proportion of lower birth weight and a decrease in the proportion of higher birth weight babies, although the relationships were slightly less marked in the group that was subsequently breast-fed.

**Table 9.4** Cohort smoking profiles of mothers who smoked at all in samples used for examining associations with pregnancy/birth, and 5/10 year outcome variables

|  | % giving up during pregnancy | Smoking through pregnancy (%) | | | $n$ (100%) |
|  |  | 1–4/day | 5–14/day | > 15/day |  |
| --- | --- | --- | --- | --- | --- |
| Sample for the study of pregnancy/birth outcomes* |  |  |  |  |  |
| Breast-feeders | 15.5 | 22.6 | 40.1 | 21.7 | 865 |
| Bottle-feeders | 8.8 | 13.1 | 47.8 | 30.3 | 3630 |
| Sample for the study of five-/10-year outcomes† |  |  |  |  |  |
| Breast-feeders | 9.8 | 20.9 | 42.7 | 26.6 | 593 |
| Bottle-feeders | 5.8 | 10.4 | 49.3 | 34.3 | 2748 |

* $\chi^2(2df) = 69.02$; $P < 0.0001$
† $\chi^2(2df) = 57.51$; $P < 0.0001$

**Table 9.5** Adjusted odds ratio of obstetric events in mothers who smoked compared with those who did not smoke in groups who subsequently breast- or bottle-fed

| Variable | Bottle/ Breast | AOR | 99% CL | Chi$^2$ | P | n1 | n2 |
|---|---|---|---|---|---|---|---|
| **Pregnancy** | | | | | | | |
| Highest | Bottle | 0.64 | 0.49–0.84 | 18.59 | <0.0001 | 472 | 5068 |
| diastolic | Breast | 0.57 | 0.34–0.94 | 8.91 | 0.0028 | 157 | 2272 |
| BP > 100 mmHg | | | | | | | |
| **Labour and delivery** | | | | | | | |
| Induced | Bottle | 0.75 | 0.64–0.89 | 19.60 | <0.0001 | 1487 | 4203 |
| delivery | Breast | 0.73 | 0.55–0.95 | 9.28 | 0.0023 | 617 | 1840 |
| Meconium | Bottle | 1.25 | 1.00–1.57 | 6.78 | 0.0092 | 636 | 4908 |
| | Breast | 1.38 | 0.98–1.95 | 5.82 | 0.0159 | 280 | 2137 |
| Birth weight | Bottle | 0.52 | 0.41–0.65 | 57.55 | <0.0001 | 707 | 5010 |
| > 3898 g | Breast | 0.68 | 0.47–0.98 | 7.67 | 0.0056 | 315 | 2157 |
| Birth weight | Bottle | 1.79 | 1.30–2.44 | 23.79 | <0.0001 | 335 | 5382 |
| < 2538 g | Breast | 1.53 | 0.85–2.75 | 3.49 | 0.0617 | 88 | 2384 |

AOR, adjusted odds ratio; CL, confidence limits; n1, number in outcome category group; n2, number in outcome contrast group.

Higher blood pressure and induction of delivery were less likely in women who smoked in each feeding group. Meconium-stained liquor was significantly more common in the smoking mothers in each feeding group, although this was most marked in mothers who later breast-fed their baby.

In general the results examined at this time indicate similar associations with maternal smoking, with a slightly reduced odds of deviant birth weights in the group of mothers later to breast-feed their child for at least a month.

## Associations with events by 5 years of age

From a total of 39 clinical and physical, health, and developmental variables reported when the children were 5 years old, nine associations with maternal smoking met the significance criteria for inclusion in Table 9.6. Most of these data derived from the mother's assessment of her child during an interview with the health visitor.

The children of smokers from both infant feeding groups were equally more likely to have been admitted to hospital during the past 5 years and to have some form of physical or mental handicap. Breast-fed children of smokers were at least as likely (if not more likely) than the bottle-fed group to have

**Table 9.6** Adjusted odds ratio of childrens' health and development at 5 years in mothers who smoked compared with those who did not smoke in groups who were subsequently breast- or bottle-fed

| Variable | Bottle/Breast | AOR | 99% CL | Chi$^2$ | P | n1 | n2 |
|---|---|---|---|---|---|---|---|
| Hospital | Bottle | 1.47 | 1.20–1.79 | 25.67 | <0.0001 | 1078 | 2964 |
| inpatient | Breast | 1.50 | 1.06–2.11 | 9.29 | 0.0023 | 361 | 1318 |
| Discharge | Bottle | 1.66 | 1.24–2.21 | 21.45 | <0.0001 | 428 | 3472 |
| from ear | Breast | 0.95 | 0.60–1.52 | 0.06 | 0.8095 | 185 | 1434 |
| Snoring | Bottle | 1.56 | 1.25–1.94 | 27.38 | <0.0001 | 789 | 3124 |
| | Breast | 1.24 | 0.87–1.77 | 2.51 | 0.1130 | 323 | 1312 |
| Bronchitis | Bottle | 1.52 | 1.21–1.92 | 23.04 | <0.0001 | 717 | 3205 |
| | Breast | 1.39 | 0.92–2.08 | 4.36 | 0.0367 | 233 | 1398 |
| Wheezing | Bottle | 1.48 | 1.20–1.83 | 23.82 | <0.0001 | 887 | 3117 |
| | Breast | 1.23 | 0.85–1.76 | 2.14 | 0.1431 | 320 | 1345 |
| Glasses | Bottle | 2.16 | 1.37–3.40 | 20.60 | <0.0001 | 174 | 3862 |
| prescribed | Breast | 2.41 | 1.16–4.98 | 9.53 | 0.0020 | 60 | 1615 |
| Ever had | Bottle | 1.54 | 1.11–2.12 | 12.30 | 0.0005 | 329 | 3681 |
| squint | Breast | 1.71 | 0.99–2.95 | 6.44 | 0.0111 | 114 | 1547 |
| Physical or mental | Bottle | 1.63 | 1.15–2.32 | 13.41 | 0.0003 | 280 | 3571 |
| handicap | Breast | 1.79 | 0.94–3.40 | 5.24 | 0.0221 | 80 | 1518 |
| IQ subnormal | Bottle | 1.61 | 1.07–2.44 | 9.17 | 0.0025 | 222 | 3621 |
| (health visitor) | Breast | 2.44 | 1.00–6.25 | 6.59 | 0.0102 | 39 | 1571 |

AOR, adjusted odds ratio; CL, confidence limits; n1, number in outcome category group; n2, number in outcome contrast group.

had a prescription for glasses or to have had a squint diagnosed in the preceding 5 years.

The results for respiratory morbidity, however, are distinct in the two infant feeding groups. Although there is a strong tendency for respiratory conditions to be significantly associated with maternal smoking, the chances of the children of smokers having a history of ear discharge, snoring or mouth breathing, wheezing, and bronchitis were markedly lower in the breast-fed than in the bottle-fed group. Of at least equal importance seems to be the association of maternal smoking in the breast-fed group with the health visitor's opinion of the child's IQ as normal or below normal. This showed that the chances of being classified as intellectually subnormal in the breast-fed children of mothers who smoked were greater than in the corresponding bottle-fed children.

## Associations at 10 years of age

Full details of the wide examination of associations between maternal smoking in pregnancy and measures of physical and intellectual development, behaviour, medical history, medical conditions, and educational achievements reported by 10 years of age are presented elsewhere (Pollock and Evans, 1991). The results presented in Table 9.7 relate only to those three areas identified to be of interest at the 5 year time point, i.e. vision, respiratory morbidity, and educational/intellectual achievement.

The chances of having had an operation for squint in the 10 years were more than doubled in the smoking group, irrespective of the method of infant feeding.

Conversely, the raised chances in the children of smokers, of a history of wheezing, bronchitis, and habitual coughing in the day or night were signi-

**Table 9.7** Adjusted odds ratio of childrens' health and development at 10 years in mothers who smoked compared with those who did not smoke in groups who were subsequently breast- or bottle-fed

| Variable | Bottle/ Breast | AOR | 99% CL | Chi$^2$ | $P$ | $n1$ | $n2$ |
|---|---|---|---|---|---|---|---|
| **Vision and respiratory complaints** | | | | | | | |
| Operation for | Bottle | 2.48 | 1.34–4.57 | 15.90 | 0.0001 | 95 | 3481 |
| squint | Breast | 2.39 | 1.85–6.80 | 4.47 | 0.0344 | 28 | 1473 |
| Wheezing history | Bottle | 1.46 | 1.16–1.83 | 19.22 | <0.0001 | 758 | 2771 |
| | Breast | 1.30 | 0.89–1.90 | 3.30 | 0.0691 | 292 | 1192 |
| Bronchitis | Bottle | 1.56 | 1.21–1.99 | 21.96 | <0.0001 | 609 | 2879 |
| history | Breast | 1.19 | 0.77–1.84 | 1.16 | 0.2820 | 212 | 1257 |
| Usually cough in | Bottle | 1.43 | 1.04–1.96 | 8.70 | 0.0032 | 343 | 3133 |
| day/night | Breast | 1.21 | 0.70–2.11 | 0.84 | 0.3590 | 118 | 1340 |
| Bronchitis in last | Bottle | 1.62 | 1.00–2.61 | 7.06 | 0.0079 | 143 | 3421 |
| year | Breast | 0.99 | 0.43–2.27 | 0.00 | 0.9751 | 52 | 1446 |
| **Educational achievement** | | | | | | | |
| Pictorial language comprehension test score greater than cohort mean | | | | | | | |
| | Bottle | 0.80 | 0.66–0.98 | 7.61 | 0.0058 | 1359 | 1875 |
| | Breast | 0.93 | 0.67–1.30 | 0.26 | 0.6099 | 795 | 542 |
| Friendly maths test score greater than cohort mean | | | | | | | |
| | Bottle | 0.77 | 0.62–0.94 | 11.11 | 0.0009 | 1600 | 1626 |
| | Breast | 0.65 | 0.46–0.91 | 10.27 | 0.0013 | 852 | 484 |
| Edinburgh reading test score greater than cohort mean | | | | | | | |
| | Bottle | 0.70 | 0.57–0.86 | 19.63 | <0.0001 | 1512 | 1723 |
| | Breast | 0.65 | 0.46–0.91 | 10.28 | 0.0013 | 854 | 485 |
| British ability scale total score greater than cohort mean | | | | | | | |
| | Bottle | 0.75 | 0.61–0.93 | 12.00 | 0.0005 | 1497 | 1667 |
| | Breast | 0.78 | 0.54–1.11 | 3.23 | 0.0723 | 872 | 446 |

AOR, adjusted odds ratio; CL, confidence limits; $n1$, number in outcome category group; $n2$, number in outcome contrast group.

ficant in the bottle-fed but not in the breast-fed group. A raised risk of bronchitis in the previous year was associated with smoking only in the bottle-fed group.

In contrast to this are the results for educational achievement as assessed by comprehension, mathematics, reading, and general intelligence tests conducted at school. The results here indicate that poorer educational achievement is associated with maternal smoking in the bottle-fed group to the same or to a greater degree as in the breast-fed group.

## Discussion

The results of this brief resumé of maternal smoking in pregnancy and various indices of adverse child health and development at 5 and 10 years of age (Evans 1989), suggest that areas of interaction with infant feeding can be proposed. The evidence is that associations between maternal smoking and respiratory morbidity interact with method of infant feeding, i.e. reduced association in breast-fed group, whereas associations with visual problems, especially that of squint, and educational achievement, seem to be largely independent of feeding method, or (with the exception of the Pictorial Language Comprehension test), are possibly even slightly exacerbated in the breast-feeding group. Further research is indicated using more precise measures of smoking and feeding obtained prospectively, together with objective assessments of outcome.

The lower magnitude of associations between maternal pregnancy/post-natal smoking and maternally reported measures of respiratory morbidity in the children of breast-feeding mothers requires explanation. One possibility is that it is a simple dose–response relationship attributable to the lower smoking rates of breast-feeding women or, alternatively, that breast-feeding itself protects against these sequelae. As neither short-term nor prolonged breast-feeding was found to have strongly significant associations with respiratory disease in this cohort after adjustment for confounding (Pollock 1991; Pollock and Evans 1991) the former explanation may be more plausible. A third possibility is that an interaction of unknown mechanism exists, in which the effect of smoking is mitigated to a degree by breast-feeding.

Conversely, sequelae of maternal smoking relating to visual problems, especially squint, and educational ability, are at least as strong or stronger in the breast-fed group. These results may indicate no interactive effect or, considering the dosage differences, can be viewed as consistent with a modest synergistic interaction between smoking and breast-feeding.

The evident possibility that the mechanism for this finding is ingestion by the infant of breast-milk contaminated by tobacco metabolites is not proven. Nicotine and cotinine concentrations in the serum of nursing smokers are in a linear relation to those in the breast-milk (Luck and Nau 1984) whilst the babies' urine cotinine levels were found by Woodward *et al.* (1986) to have a linear relationship with the mothers' smoking rates in breast-fed, but not in wholly bottle-fed, 3-month-old infants. The latter result is of particular interest, as breast-feeding smokers smoked less and reported greater smoking 'hygiene', i.e. not smoking in the same room as the infant, compared to the bottle-feeding mothers. Similar results have more recently been reported by Labrecque *et al.* (1989), and it seems probable that breast-milk is the main source of cotinine and nicotine in infants of breast-feeding smoking mothers.

In conclusion, the hypothesis that smoking by the mother in pregnancy can itself influence lactation or breast-feeding ability is not refuted by an examination of the literature or by new epidemiological analyses. Furthermore, the second hypothesis, that interactions exist between smoking and infant feeding in some long-term sequelae of maternal smoking is supported by an analysis of data from longitudinal studies of children in the 1970 British Births Survey. The epidemiological evidence is not sufficiently precise to suggest possible aetiological pathways but further research activity in this area is clearly indicated. This conclusion is of topical concern as health messages to promote breast-feeding have been much more successful than those discouraging smoking in women of child-bearing age.

# References

Andersen, A. N., Lund-Andersen, C., Larsen, J. F., Christensen, N. J., Legros, J. J., Louis, F., *et al.* (1982). Suppressed prolactin but normal neurophysin levels in cigarette smoking breast-feeding women. *Clinical Endocrinology,* **17,** 363–8.

Andersen, A. N., Ronn, B., Tjonneland, A., Djursing, H., and Schioler, V. (1984). Low maternal but normal foetal prolactin levels in cigarette smoking pregnant women. *Acta Obstetrica et Gynecologica Scandinavica,* **63,** 237–9.

Butler, N. R. and Golding, J. (1986). *From birth to five.* Pergamon Press, Oxford.

Chamberlain, R., Chamberlain, G., Howlett, B., and Claireaux, A. (1975). British Births 1970 Vol. 1 *The First Week of Life.* Heinemann Medical Books Ltd, London.

Cross, B. A. (1955). The hypothalamus and the mechanism of sympathetico–adreno inhibition of milk ejection. *Journal of Endocrinology,* **12,** 15–18.

Evans, J. A. (1989). Long-term associations between parental smoking and child development. In *The needs of parents and infants,* pp. 19–27. Health Promotion Research Trust, Cambridge.

Ferry, J. D., Mclean, B. K., and Winer, M. B. (1974). Tobacco smoke inhalation delays suckling-induced prolactin release in the rat. *Proceedings of the Society for Experimental Biology and Medicine,* **147,** 110–13.

Labrecque, M., Marcoux, S., Weber, J. P., Fabia, J., and Ferron, L. (1989). Feeding and urine cotinine values in babies whose mothers smoke. *Pediatrics,* **83(1),** 93–7.

Luck, W. and Nau, H. (1984). Nicotine and cotinine concentrations, in serum and milk of nursing smokers. *British Journal of Clinical Pharmacy,* **18,** 9–15.

Lyon, A. J. (1983). Effects of smoking on breast feeding. *Archives of Disease in Childhood,* **58,** 378–80.

Martin, J. and White, A. (1988). *Infant feeding 1985.* Office of Population Censuses and Surveys (Social Survey Division), HMSO, London.

Martin, D. C., Martin, J. C., and Streissguth, A. P. (1979). Smoking frequency and amplitude in newborns as a function of maternal drinking and smoking. In *Currents in alcoholism,* (ed. M. Galanter), pp. 359–66. Grune and Stratton Inc, London.

Nylander, G. and Matheson, I. (1989). Breast-feeding. Effects of smoking and education. *Tidsskrift Nor Laegeforen,* **109(9),** 970–3. (Abstract only seen.)

Office of Population Censuses and Surveys (OPCS) (1988). *OPCS Monitor,* 9 February.

Pollock, J. I. (1991). *Continuing to Breast-Feed,* Report, Health Promotion Research Trust, no. 6.

Pollock, J. I. and Evans, J. A. (1991). *Parental Smoking,* Report, Health Promotion Research Trust, no. 2.

Pollock, J. I. and Thomas, (1991). *Starting to Breast-Feed,* Report, Health Promotion Research Trust, no. 5.

Said, G., Patois, E., and Lellouch, J. (1984). Infantile colic and parental smoking. *British Medical Journal,* **259,** 680.

Topping, D. L. (1980). Effects of tobacco smoke and its constituents on lipid and carbohydrate metabolism. In *Biochemistry of cellular regulation, vol. II: Clinical and scientific aspects of regulation of metabolism,* (ed. M. J. Clemens and M. Ashwell), pp. 165–83. CRC Press, Boca Raton, Florida.

Whichelow, M. J. and King, B. E. (1979). Breast-feeding and smoking. *Archives of Disease in Childhood,* **54,** 240–1.

Woodward, A. and Hand, K. (1988). Smoking and reduced duration of breast-feeding. *Medical Journal of Australia,* **148(2),** 477–8.

Woodward, A., Grgurinovich, N., and Ryan, P. (1986). Breast-feeding and smoking hygiene. *Journal of Epidemiology and Community Health,* **40,** 309–15.

Yeung, D. L., Penndl, M. D., Leung, M., and Hall, J. (1981). Effects of maternal cigarette smoking during pregnancy on birth size, growth of infants and infant feeding practices. *Nutrition Reports International,* **23(5),** 887–900.

# 10. Parental smoking and respiratory problems in childhood

*Julie-Ann Evans and Jean Golding*

## Passive smoking in childhood

There have been many studies on the possible respiratory effects of exposure to tobacco smoke during childhood. Studies with reasonably large numbers are listed in Table 10.1. There is a lack of consistency in ages, condition, type of population, and statistical methods used. Nevertheless, the vast majority of studies do find some effects of smoking. These are summarized briefly below.

Nine studies have looked at parental smoking and chronic cough in the child. Three of these found no association (Liard *et al.* 1982; Schenker *et al.* 1983; Clifford *et al.* 1989), one found an association with both parents smoking (Bland *et al.* 1978), one found an association that was due more to maternal than paternal smoking (Charlton 1984) and two found an association with the number of smokers in the household, which disappeared after controlling for adult phlegm production (Colley 1974*a*; Lebowitz and Burrows 1976). Two further studies showed an association with parental smoking when the coughs occurred together with colds (Weiss *et al.* 1980; Ekwo *et al.* 1983).

Six studies have looked at bronchitis or pneumonia in early childhood. All showed some sort of effect, but findings varied with the definition of disorder and the age of the child. For example, one study showed an association between maternal smoking and bronchitis with wheezing but not for bronchitis without wheezing (Liard *et al.* 1982). The same study showed a dose effect, in that the more cigarettes the mother smoked the more likely was the child to have wheezy bronchitis. An American study showed an association between maternal smoking and chest illness and similar associations were found whether the child's illness occurred in the first 2 years of life or when the child was at school (Schenker *et al.* 1983). The data from the Christchurch cohort in New Zealand showed a very clear association between maternal, but not paternal, smoking and bronchitis/pneumonia in the first year of life (Fergusson *et al.* 1980) but that the association was much smaller in the second year and was not present in the third year (Fergusson *et al.* 1981). Data from the Harrow prospective study also found that the association was strong for infants of under 1 year (Leeder *et al.* 1976*a*) but not consistent thereafter (Colley 1974*b*).

**Table 10.1** Literature review of passive smoking in childhood

| Author and date | Details of study |
|---|---|
| **Schenker *et al.* (1983)** | |
| Sample | USA, sample of schools, child interview and parental self-completion for children aged 5–14 ($n = 4071$) |
| Outcomes | Cough/phlegm, wheeze, chest illness, asthma |
| [1]Factors | Age, sex, socio-economic status, parental allergy, parental respiratory disease, gas cooking |
| Results | Maternal smoking associated with increase in chest illness in past year and before the age of 2. No association with cough/phlegm, wheeze or asthma |
| **Liard *et al.* (1982)** | |
| Sample | France, day nurseries, maternal interview for infants aged 6–12 months ($n = 424$) |
| Outcomes | Upper respiratory tract infection, cough, bronchitis, infant wheeze, wheezy bronchitis |
| [1]Factors | None |
| Results | No association between maternal smoking and URTI, bronchitis, infant wheeze or cough. Dose–response relationship with wheezy bronchitis (3.1%, 10.4%, 15.6% for no cigarettes, $< 20$, $20+$ respectively) $P < 0.0005$ |
| **Clifford *et al.* (1989)** | |
| Sample | Southampton school children aged 7 and 11 ($n = 2503$) |
| Outcomes | Wheeze, cough, shortness of breath |
| [1]Factors | None |
| Results | No association with parental smoking |
| **Bland *et al.* (1978)** | |
| Sample | Derbyshire, secondary school cross-section ($n = 6330$) |
| Outcomes | Cough, breathlessness |
| [1]Factors | Sex, child's smoking |
| Results | Relative risks (M, F) for both parents smoking compared with neither: cough in morning (1.4, 2.0), cough during day or night (1.4, 1.5), breathlessness (1.4, 1.3) |
| **Charlton (1984)** | |
| Sample | Northern England, stratified sample of school questionnaires to children aged 8–19 ($n = 15126$) |
| Outcomes | 'Do you get a lot of coughs?' |
| [1]Factors | Social area, child's smoking, age, sex, region |
| Results | Trend with the number of parents smoking. Mothers smoking more influence than fathers |
| **Colley (1974*a*)** | |
| Sample | Aylesbury (UK) school children aged 6–14, parental self-completion ($n = 2426$) |

**Table 10.1** (*Continued*)

---

| | |
|---|---|
| Outcomes | Cough |
| [1]Factors | Number of sibling, social class |
| Results | Gradient in prevalence according to number of parents smoking but totally due to association with phlegm |

Lebowitz and Burrows (1976)

| | |
|---|---|
| Sample | USA, stratified sample, parental questionnaire for children < 15 (*n* = 626) |
| Outcomes | Cough, phlegm, wheeze |
| [1]Factors | Age, social status, family size |
| Results | Higher rates of persistent cough for children in houses with adult smokers. Significance lost if control for adult symptoms |

Ekwo *et al.* (1983)

| | |
|---|---|
| Sample | USA, parental self-completion, primary school children aged 6–12 (*n* = 1355) |
| Outcomes | Cough, hospital admission for respiratory illness |
| [1]Factors | Gas cooking |
| Results | Odds ratios: wheezing with cold, 1.3; cough with cold, 1.5; hospital admission for respiratory problem, 2.1 |

Weiss *et al.* (1980)

| | |
|---|---|
| Sample | USA, school-children aged 5–9, parental interview and fortnightly telephone for 2 years (*n* = 650) |
| Outcomes | Acute respiratory illness, croup, bronchitis, pneumonia, cough, phlegm, wheeze, infant colds, asthma, lung function (FEV) |
| [1]Factors | Parental phlegm and wheeze, asthma, child's smoking |
| Results | Trend for wheeze, cough and phlegm with the number of parents smoking. FEV was related to maternal but not paternal smoking |

Fergusson *et al.* (1980)

| | |
|---|---|
| Sample | New Zealand, prospective population studied at 0, 4 months & 12 months (*n* = 1180) |
| Outcomes | Medical consultation for bronchitis, bronchitis or pneumonia, wheezy chest |
| [1]Factors | Birth weight, gestation, maternal age and education, race, family size, living standards, breast-feeding |
| Results | Maternal smoking, but not paternal smoking associated with increased consultation for, and symptoms of lower respiratory tract infection, and with reduced symptoms of upper respiratory tract infection |

Fergusson *et al.* (1981)

| | |
|---|---|
| Sample | New Zealand, prospective population, first 3 years (*n* = 1265) |
| Outcomes | Bronchitis, pneumonia, symptoms of wheezy chest |
| [1]Factors | Maternal age and education, family size, living standards |
| Results | Maternal smoking positively associated with respiratory problem in the first year, smaller association for problems in the 2nd year, no association with 3rd year. No paternal smoking effect |

**Table 10.1** (*Continued*)

| Author and date | Details |
| --- | --- |

**Leeder *et al.* (1976*a*)**

| | |
| --- | --- |
| Sample | Harrow, geographic population of up to 1 year ($n = 2205$) |
| Outcomes | Lower respiratory tract infection |
| [1]Factors | Number of siblings, parental cough or phlegm and asthma or wheeze, sibling bronchitis or pneumonia |
| Results | Trend for bronchitis or pneumonia with number of parents smoking. Adjusted incidence rates 6.2, 9.7, 15.4 for neither parent smoked, one smoked, both smoked respectively ($P < 0.0005$) |

**Colley (1974*b*)**

| | |
| --- | --- |
| Sample | Harrow, geographic population up to 5 years ($n = 2205$) |
| Outcomes | Bronchitis, pneumonia |
| [1]Factors | Social class, number of siblings, parental phlegm, birth weight |
| Results | Association with smoking for problems in 1st year but not consistent for problem after 1 year |

**Hosein *et al.* (1989)**

| | |
| --- | --- |
| Sample | USA girls aged 7–14 and boys aged 7–17 ($n = 729 + 628$) |
| Outcomes | FEV, reported current cough, phlegm, wheeze, dyspnoea |
| [1]Factors | Air conditioning, gas cooking, crowding |
| Results | Trend for wheeze, but not FEV, with number of parents smoking. No dose effect |

**Gortmaker *et al.* (1982)**

| | |
| --- | --- |
| Sample | USA, children 0–17 in 1 high- and 1 low-prevalence area, parental self-completion ($n = 3072 + 894$) |
| Outcomes | Reported asthma, functional impairment due to asthma |
| [1]Factors | Hayfever, other allergies, maternal education, family income, age, sex |
| Results | Maternal smoking, but not paternal, significantly associated with both outcomes. Odds ratios in two areas 1.5 and 1.8 for asthma, 2.0 and 2.4 for impairment |

**Lucas *et al.* (1990)**

| | |
| --- | --- |
| Sample | Cambridge (UK), 5-centre hospital births $< 1850$ g ($n = 777$) |
| Outcomes | Recurrent wheeze or asthma |
| [1]Factors | Sex, birth weight, small-for-gestational age, gestation, mode of delivery, ventilation, pre-eclampsia, intra-uterine growth retardation, social class, family history of allergy |
| Results | Positive, dose-related association with maternal smoking. No effect of paternal smoking |

**Leeder *et al.* (1976*b*)**

| | |
| --- | --- |
| Sample | Harrow, prospective population up to 5 years ($n = 1878$) |
| Outcomes | Asthma or wheeze |
| [1]Factors | Sex, bronchitis or pneumonia in 1st year, parental cough or phlegm |
| Results | Increased rates of wheezing for parental smoking but not significant after adjusting. No association with asthma |

**Table 10.1** (*Continued*)

---

Tager *et al.* (1979)
    Sample     USA, school-children 5–9 years, parental interview (*n* = 444)
    Outcomes  Lung function
    [1]Factors   None
    Results    Reduced lung function (FEV) with number of smoking
               parents

Berkey *et al.* (1986)
    Sample     East and mid-West USA school-children (non-smoking) aged
               6–18 (*n* = 7834)
    Outcomes  Lung function (FEV, FVC) (age 8) and growth rates
    [1]Factors   City, parental education, height, weight, sex, age
    Results    Maternal smoking associated with both FEV measures, not with FVC
               and slightly with FVC growth. No paternal smoking effect

Tager *et al.* (1983)
    Sample     USA children aged 5–9 followed for 7-year interviews (*n* = 1156)
    Outcomes  Respiratory symptoms, lung function (FEV)
    [1]Factors   Age, sex, height, maternal education, gas cooking
    Results    Maternal smoking associated with FEV. No paternal smoking
               effect

Chen and Li (1986)
    Sample     China, school-children aged 8–16 years (*n* = 571)
    Outcomes  Lung function (FVC, FEV, MMEF, FEF)
    [1]Factors   Age, height, weight, paternal education, gas cooking, area
    Results    Paternal smoking linearly associated with FEV, MMEF, FEF. Larger
               effect for girls than boys

Iversen *et al.* (1985)
    Sample     Denmark, children in day care aged 0–7, fortnightly tympanometry for
               3 months
    Outcomes  Middle ear effusion
    [1]Factors   Number of children in institution, number of siblings, housing, age
    Results    Association with parental association (odds ratio 1.6)

Said *et al.* (1978)
    Sample     Paris, secondary school, pupils aged 10–20 (*n* = 3920)
    Outcomes  Tonsillectomy and/or adenoidectomy
    [1]Factors   Age, sex, number of siblings, day nursery attendance
    Results    Independent associations with maternal and paternal smoking

Vogt (1984)
    Sample     Oregon, USA, insurance population, parental interview for children
               aged 0–18 (*n* = 1761)
    Outcomes  Doctor/outpatient visits for respiratory conditions
    [1]Factors   Age, number of children, socio-economic status
    Results    No association with parental smoking

**Table 10.1** (*Continued*)

| Author and date | Details |
|---|---|
| | |

**Bonham and Wilson (1982)**

| | |
|---|---|
| Sample | USA, stratified sample, National Health interview. Number not stated |
| [1]Factors | Days of restricted activity, bed disability due to acute illness |
| [1]Factors | Age, number of adults, income, education of head of household |
| Results | Number of smoking adults and number of cigarettes smoked showed trend with restricted activity due to respiratory illness |

**Ogston *et al.* (1985)**

| | |
|---|---|
| Sample | Tayside, population of primigravidae followed for 1 year ($n = 1565$) |
| Outcomes | Health Visitor record of respiratory illness, hospital admission for respiratory illness |
| [1]Factors | Type of heating, cooking, maternal age, breast-feeding |
| Results | Positive association for smoking of either parent with both outcomes |

**Chen *et al.* (1986)**

| | |
|---|---|
| Sample | Shanghai, China, population, self-completion questionnaire ($n = 1058$) |
| Outcomes | Hospital admission for respiratory illness $< 18$ months |
| [1]Factors | Sex, twin, breast-feeding, birth weight, paternal education, maternal age, coal cooking, crowding, income, household, respiratory disease |
| Results | Paternal smoking dose–response effect |

[1] Refers to factors taken into account.

Nine reports studied wheezing and/or asthma. Seven showed significant associations with parental smoking:

(1) wheeze with parental smoking (Hosein *et al.* 1989);
(2) asthma with maternal, but not paternal, smoking (Gortmaker *et al.* 1982);
(3) recurrent wheeze or asthma with maternal, but not paternal, smoking (Lucas *et al.* 1990);
(4) a wheezy chest in the first year of life with maternal smoking (Fergusson *et al.* 1980);
(5) a wheezing association with parental smoking only if the wheeze was accompanied by a cold (Ekwo *et al.* 1983);
(6) an association between wheezing and parental smoking that disappeared once parental cough, phlegm, and bronchitis/pneumonia had been taken into account (the Harrow study, Leeder *et al.* 1976*b*);
(7) an association between recurrent wheeze and maternal smoking even when these factors were controlled for (Weiss *et al.* 1980).

Lung function tests have been carried out in six different studies. Only one showed no association with parental smoking (Hosein *et al.* 1989). One study showed abnormalities in lung function related to both maternal and paternal smoking (Tager *et al.* 1979); three showed a relationship with maternal, but not paternal, smoking (Tager *et al.* 1983; Weiss *et al.* 1980; Berkey *et al.* 1986); and one showed a relationship with paternal, but not maternal, smoking (Chen and Li 1986). The latter study was in China, where it is very rare for a mother to smoke.

As far as upper respiratory tract infections are concerned, one study showed no effect with parental smoking (Liard *et al.* 1982) and in one there was a negative effect (Fergusson *et al.* 1980). When considering specifically middle ear effusions, however, parental smoking had a positive association (Iversen *et al.* 1985) and associations were also found with frequency of tonsillectomy and/or adenoidectomy (Said *et al.* 1978).

Studies that did not distinguish between upper and lower respiratory conditions include general practitioner visits for respiratory conditions (no effect, Vogt 1984) and number of days of restricted activity because of respiratory problems (positive association with the number of smoking adults and the dose of cigarettes smoked in the home (Bonham and Wilson 1982). There have been three studies looking at early hospitalization for respiratory conditions (Ekwo *et al.* 1983; Ogston *et al.* 1985; Chen *et al.* 1986). All show positive effects with parental smoking, although it should be noted that in China, again, there was only an effect with paternal smoking as mothers did not smoke (Chen *et al.* 1986).

The majority of the studies in Table 10.1 were cross-sectional in nature and considered the current smoking habit of the parents together with the current symptoms or the past history of the child. No account was taken of parental smoking habits during pregnancy and hence of fetal exposure. There have, however, been six studies which have looked at the relationship between pregnancy smoking and childhood respiratory problems.

## Fetal exposure to maternal smoking in pregnancy

In Israel, antenatal information on maternal smoking was linked prospectively to the hospital records of 10 672 children. For those admitted in the first year with upper respiratory tract infections, there was no association with maternal smoking in pregnancy, but admissions for bronchitis or pneumonia were positively associated, even after controlling for birth weight, social class, and birth order. Women who had been smokers before pregnancy but not during pregnancy showed no relationship with this outcome. Among mothers who had smoked throughout pregnancy there was a dose–response effect in that the more cigarettes smoked the greater the likelihood for the child to have been admitted with a lower respiratory infection. There was also an age effect, with the strongest smoking association seen for admissions for bronchitis and pneumonia between 6 and 9 months of age (Harlap and Davies 1974).

Chan and colleagues (1989*a, b*) prospectively followed a small number of low birth weight (less than 2000 g) children to the age of seven. This London hospital population was then given lung function tests and, after allowing for sex, height, ethnic group, and neonatal treatment a reduction associated with maternal smoking in pregnancy was shown in the maximum expiratory flow. There was no association with smoking by other household members. Answers to self-completion questionnaires by 121 of the parents of these children revealed an association between a history of wheeze and of cough and maternal smoking in pregnancy, even after controlling for social class, neonatal oxygen treatment, a family history of asthma, and a skin test for atopy. The association with wheeze was particularly strong (odds ratio (OR) 3.39; 95 per cent confidence interval (CI) 1.13–10.2).

In Denmark, 5953 hospital births were followed for the first year of life (Bisgaard *et al.* 1987). A history of wheezing (excluding that due to pneumonia, epiglottitis, and acute laryngitis) was associated strongly with maternal smoking during pregnancy ($P < 0.001$) even after controlling for social status and sex.

In Finland 1819 mothers who smoked during pregnancy were identified from a series of 12 068 mothers studied initially during the sixth and seventh months of pregnancy (Rantakallio 1983). Controls were selected and matched for the number of children born, marital status, age, parity, and place of residence of the mother and were followed up to the age of 14 with data on hospital admissions up to 10 years of age. The children of smokers had more frequent hospital admissions for respiratory diseases, both up to 5 years and between 5 and 10 years of age ($P = 0.024$). At the age of 14 the population with asthma was the same in both groups (2.1 per cent), but the children of smokers had slightly higher (not statistically significant) rates of admission for asthma.

The biggest longitudinal study was the National Child Development Study, which followed 8641 children prospectively from birth up to the age of 16. Parental questionnaires at 16 identified those children who had had asthma or wheezy bronchitis at any stage. There was a strong association between such a history and the maternal history of smoking heavily in pregnancy, but after controlling for sex, birth weight, gestation, parity, social class, and maternal age the group of children of moderate smokers were shown to have reduced prevalence of such a history (Fogelman 1980). There were interactions with gestation, birth weight, and maternal age that caused the authors to be somewhat sceptical about long-term associations.

## Problems in interpretation

In many of the above studies there has often been a tendency to over-control.

For example, to look at maternal smoking and control for birth weight and gestation (Fogelman 1980; Lucas *et al.* 1990), or examine childhood wheezing and control for parental respiratory disease (Leeder *et al.* 1976*a, b*; Schenker *et al.* 1983) is over-controlling and artificially diminishing any association that may be present.

Although, with the exception of the data from China, the balance of results indicate that it is maternal smoking that is associated with childhood respiratory disorder, none of the studies quoted has information on both antenatal and postnatal exposure. There is currently only one data set with the information necessary for this analysis: the 1970 British Births Cohort (Butler and Golding 1986).

There have been a number of studies using these data, both cross-sectionally and longitudinally. A cross-sectional study at 5 years of age showed statistically significant associations between maternal smoking at that age and a history in the children of wheezing, bronchitis, pneumonia, ear discharge, and mouth breathing or snoring (Butler and Golding 1986). In 1989 Neuspiel and colleagues looked at parental smoking throughout the first 10 years of life, but took no account of smoking in pregnancy. They showed a 14 per cent increase in incidence of wheezy bronchitis when the mother smoked 5–14 cigarettes per day, and a 49 per cent increase for children of mothers who smoked 15 or more cigarettes per day. The only previously published study of these data took account of both prenatal and postnatal exposure and showed that hospital admission for lower respiratory tract illness before the age of 5 was related to pregnancy rather than postnatal smoking and that reported bronchitis before the age of 5 was probably influenced by both prenatal and postnatal effects, but the prenatal effect was strongest (Taylor and Wadsworth 1987).

This chapter reports the results of new analyses of these data using a different methodology, which confirms and extends the conclusions of Taylor and Wadsworth (1987).

## The 1970 Birth Cohort Study

For 98.5 per cent of all women delivering a live child or a stillbirth in Great Britain in the week 5–11 April 1970, midwives filled in questionnaires relating to the history of pregnancy and delivery, demographic characteristics, and health behaviour, including smoking history during pregnancy (Chamberlain *et al.* 1975, 1978). When the children were aged 5, some 80 per cent were traced and mothers completed questionnaires administered by health visitors. The questions involved details of the current smoking habits of both parents, any history of wheezing, and its frequency, any history of bronchitis, pneumonia, and upper respiratory problems such as frequent sore throats requiring medical attention, ear discharge (pus not wax), and habitual mouth breathing or snoring (Butler and Golding 1986). In 1980, a new attempt was made to trace all of the children in the birth cohort. In the event, some 94 per cent were identified and mothers were again interviewed. Once again, the mothers responded to questions on frequency of wheezing, history of bronchitis and pneumonia, and frequency of coughing. The child was also asked about shortness of breath when hurrying.

## Statistical methodology

To determine the effects of smoking independent of factors predictive of smoking, a methodology was developed that identified first all those independent environmental, social, and medical factors that predicted a mother smoking. Then, taking these factors into account, the independent effect of smoking on the outcome under consideration was determined.

For the present analyses, three different models were studied. First, to determine the possible effects of smoking in pregnancy, all 7429 (46 per cent) such mothers were compared with all 8692 (54 per cent) mothers who did not smoke in pregnancy. The predictive factors were identified and then the outcomes were studied. Because some of the predictive factors depended on past obstetric history, primigravidae and multigravidae were considered separately. Secondly, to determine the effect of smoking after delivery, all 918 (14 per cent) mothers who did not smoke in pregnancy, but who smoked subsequently were compared with all 5626 (86 per cent) mothers who never smoked at all either during pregnancy or later in the child's life. Lastly, to assess the effects of giving up smoking in pregnancy, the 764 mothers who fell into this category were compared with those 6665 who smoked throughout and with those 8692 who never smoked.

## Results

Table 10.2 gives the results for maternal smoking during pregnancy in relation to respiratory outcomes.

For primiparae, there was a 23–27 per cent increase in the risk of wheezing and of bronchitis in their children, whether measured at 5 or 10 years. These associations were statistically significant. There were also increased odds ratios for a history of pneumonia by 5 and by 10, but the numbers were not large enough for statistical significance. At the age of 5 the association with risk of habitual mouth breathing or snoring and of ear discharge was higher and more statistically significant than those with wheezing and bronchitis. However, by the age of 10, there was no association with cough or shortness of breath.

The same associations were seen among multiparae. It can be seen from Table 10.2 that the odds ratios for the risk of bronchitis and of pneumonia were higher for multiparae who smoked in pregnancy than for primiparae, although the odds of wheezing were similar. The relationships with habitual snoring/mouth breathing and ear discharge were also similar in primiparae

**Table 10.2** Respiratory outcomes of children of mothers smoking in pregnancy compared with mothers who did not smoke in pregnancy

|  | Adjusted odds ratio (95% CI) | |
|---|---|---|
|  | Parity 0 | Parity 1+ |
| History of wheezing by 5 years | 1.23 (1.05–1.44)* | 1.38 (1.22–1.55)*** |
| History of wheezing by 10 years | 1.24 (1.06–1.45)** | 1.26 (1.12–1.43)*** |
| History of bronchitis by 5 years | 1.27 (1.06–1.52)** | 1.53 (1.34–1.72)*** |
| History of bronchitis by 10 years | 1.26 (1.07–1.50)** | 1.60 (1.39–1.82)*** |
| History of pneumonia by 5 years | 1.50 (0.83–2.69) | 2.10 (1.41–3.13)*** |
| History of pneumonia by 10 years | 1.39 (0.88–2.20) | 1.64 (1.16–2.33)** |
| Habitual snoring/mouth breathing at 5 years | 1.35 (1.16–1.58)*** | 1.31 (1.15–1.39)*** |
| History of ear discharge (pus not wax) at 5 years | 1.34 (1.10–1.64)** | 1.33 (1.14–1.56)*** |
| Sore throats at 5 years | 1.07 (0.92–1.24) | 1.03 (0.91–1.17) |
| Cough at 10 years | 1.13 (0.93–1.37) | 1.26 (1.07–1.43)** |
| Shortness of breath at 10 years | 0.94 (0.81–1.10) | 1.22 (1.08–1.37)** |

* $P < 0.05$; ** $P < 0.01$; *** $P < 0.001$.

and multiparae. However, children of multiparae, but not primiparae, had increased odds of cough at the age of 10 and shortness of breath.

Table 10.3 shows that postnatal smoking by mothers who had not smoked in pregnancy was not associated with an increased risk of subequent wheezing in the child. Nevertheless, there was some indication that the passive postnatal smoking was related to an increased risk of bronchitis, although this failed to reach statistical significance. No relationships with pneumonia were discernible, but those with habitual snoring/mouth breathing and ear discharge were very similar to those found for pregnancy smoking. In addition, the relationship with cough at 10 years was very similar to that found for multiparae who smoked in pregnancy. There was no relationship, however, with shortness of breath at 10 years of age.

If smoking during pregnancy is really the most important feature, it is pertinent to identify at what stage during pregnancy the effects take place. Table 10.4 compares the histories of children of mothers who were smoking at the beginning of pregnancy but who had stopped by the end of pregnancy with those whose mothers had smoked throughout pregnancy and those whose mothers had never smoked during pregnancy. It must be remembered that mothers who smoked throughout pregnancy tended to continue smoking postnatally and smoked more heavily than mothers who gave up during pregnancy. From the first column of the table it can be seen that there was

**Table 10.3** Respiratory outcomes of children of mothers who did not smoke in pregnancy but smoked postnatally compared with mothers who never smoked

|  | Adjusted odds ratio (95% CI) |
| --- | --- |
| History of wheezing by 5 years | 1.06 (0.88–1.27) |
| History of wheezing by 10 years | 1.03 (0.84–1.26) |
| History of bronchitis by 5 years | 1.21 (0.99–1.47) |
| History of bronchitis by 10 years | 1.13 (0.91–1.41) |
| History of pneumonia by 5 years | 0.95 (0.47–1.95) |
| History of pneumonia by 10 years | 0.90 (0.49–1.67) |
| Habitual snoring/mouth breathing at 5 years | 1.30 (1.09–1.56)** |
| History of ear discharge (pus not wax) at 5 years | 1.27 (1.01–1.59)* |
| Sore throats at 5 years | 1.21 (1.02–1.44)* |
| Cough at 10 years | 1.31 (1.03–1.67)* |
| Shortness of breath at 10 years | 1.08 (0.90–1.31) |

* $P < 0.05$; ** $P < 0.01$.

basically little difference in the respiratory outcomes of the children of the mothers who gave up and those of mothers who did not.

However, the odds ratios are, in general, less than 1, implying that those mothers who gave up during pregnancy had children at a lower risk of these conditions. Most of these mothers had stopped smoking by the end of the second trimester and thus the children were not exposed to smoke during the third trimester. Nevertheless, as already mentioned, the mothers who gave up tended to smoke fewer cigarettes than mothers who smoked throughout. It cannot be concluded with any certainty from these data, that giving up by the end of the second trimester protects the child from later disorder.

The comparison between the chances of respiratory disease in children of mothers who gave up with those whose mothers did not smoke in pregnancy again shows little in the way of statistically significant effects, except in respect of habitual snoring and mouth breathing at age 5. This association, as has already been shown, is more likely to be one of postnatal than prenatal smoke exposure. Other features of interest, however, are the increased relationship with wheezing, bronchitis, and pneumonia at the age of 10; even though these were not statistically highly significant, they are all in the same direction and indicate that mothers who were smoking in pregnancy placed their child at greater risk of long-term poor outcome.

## Discussion

The results indicate that the effects of passive smoking during the child's life

**Table 10.4** Respiratory outcomes of children of mothers who stopped smoking in pregnancy compared with children of mothers who smoked throughout and children of mothers who did not smoke in pregnancy

|  | Adjusted odds ratio (95% CI) | |
|  | Comparison with 'smoked throughout pregnancy' | Comparison with 'did not smoke in pregnancy' |
|---|---|---|
| History of wheezing by 5 years | 0.85 (0.68–1.07) | 1.05 (0.84–1.31) |
| History of wheezing by 10 years | 0.99 (0.79–1.23) | 1.17 (0.94–1.46) |
| History of bronchitis by 5 years | 0.85 (0.66–1.09) | 1.10 (0.86–1.41) |
| History of bronchitis by 10 years | 0.88 (0.69–1.12) | 1.25 (0.99–1.58) |
| History of pneumonia by 5 years | 0.59 (0.25–1.37) | 1.06 (0.45–2.48) |
| History of pneumonia by 10 years | 0.88 (0.45–1.72) | 1.51 (0.82–2.80) |
| Habitual snoring/mouth breathing at 5 years | 1.05 (0.85–1.31) | 1.46 (1.18–1.80)*** |
| History of ear discharge (pus not wax) at 5 years | 0.84 (0.63–1.12) | 1.07 (0.80–1.43) |
| Sore throats at 5 years | 1.01 (0.81–1.26) | 1.10 (0.89–1.37) |
| Cough at 10 years | 0.87 (0.65–1.17) | 1.03 (0.77–1.37) |
| Shortness of breath at 10 years | 1.06 (0.86–1.31) | 1.10 (0.89–1.45) |

*** $P < 0.001$.

are far less marked for lower respiratory conditions than they are for upper respiratory conditions. Moreover, the relationship between postnatal smoking and habitual snoring/mouth breathing and of ear discharge were similar in the three different analyses. This would indicate that postnatal smoking is the key smoking exposure rather than prenatal smoking.

For wheezing, there was no relationship with postnatal smoking but there was with prenatal smoking, implying that this is the key factor. It has certainly been found that mothers who smoke during pregnancy have infants with elevated cord blood IgE levels (Warren *et al.* 1982). This could indicate an increased allergic response, which may last throughout the child's life. If so, this might explain the wheezing association, and the fact that it seemed to be only related to prenatal smoking.

A history of bronchitis, and of pneumonia, was very strongly related to maternal smoking during pregnancy, but these mothers also smoke later during the child's life. Nevertheless, the fact that the postnatal smoking effects are much reduced for bronchitis and non-existent for pneumonia indicates that the key factor is maternal smoking during pregnancy. Here the mechanism may be very different to that shown for wheezing. Harrison

(1979) showed that there was a reduction in the total lymphocytes and neutrophils in the cord blood of babies born to heavy smokers. He stated that any agent, such as maternal smoking, which reduces the number of neutrophils in the vascular compartment will inhibit the mechanisms of resistance to infection.

The effects of bronchitis and wheezing are independent of one another. Examination of children who had both bronchitis and wheezing attacks, those who had bronchitis and never wheezed, and those who had wheezing but never bronchitis, showed all had strong relationships with maternal smoking in pregnancy. Of these, only bronchitis without wheeze showed a relationship with postnatal smoking, although this failed to reach statistical significance (OR 1.28; 95 per cent CI 0.99–1.66).

The history of bronchitis and pneumonia and its relationship with smoking was stronger for the multiparae than for primiparae. The assumption here would be that children who have older siblings are brought earlier and more frequently in contact with infections, and if the mothers had smoked in pregnancy the children would be unduly vulnerable.

Age at onset of these infections and maternal smoking has received much discussion in the literature. This data set showed that relationships with bronchitis and wheezing at the age of 10 did not totally disappear when one controlled for such a history at the age of 5. Thus the relationships with maternal history of smoking in pregnancy, although reduced for wheezing at 10, still produced odds ratios of 1.13 in children of primiparae and 1.18 in multiparae ($P = 0.06$); odds ratios for bronchitis for the two parity groups were 1.20 and 1.39, even after allowing for a history of bronchitis at the age of 5.

The implications of this are that maternal smoking in pregnancy has a prolonged effect on respiratory problems in childhood. Nevertheless, from these data it is not possible to judge whether particular age groups are more at risk than others.

## Conclusions

This chapter has shown that, as previously reported, there is a strong relationship between maternal smoking and respiratory problems in the child. The bulk of the evidence from the prospective data shows that it is maternal smoking during pregnancy that makes the child particularly vulnerable to subsequent wheezing, bronchitis, and pneumonia, but that it is postnatal smoking that makes the child vulnerable to habitual snoring/mouth breathing, ear discharge, and possibly chronic cough.

There are, however, a number of queries raised by the data as analysed here. First of all, it is not possible from the numbers available to determine whether the risks are reduced in mothers who gave up smoking during pregnancy, or whether there will be long-term effects on the lung function of these children. It has not been possible to distinguish the mothers who smoked during pregnancy but who subsequently did not smoke from those who continued to smoke throughout the child's life, as almost all who smoked throughout pregnancy continued to do so. There is some animal evidence that the effects of exposure to smoke in pregnancy may be reduced in those who are not postnatally exposed, but there is little human data to test this.

The strong associations with paternal but not maternal smoking reported from China remain unexplained. Nevertheless, it must be remembered that the cigarettes smoked in China are particularly strong and toxic. The study in Shanghai will presumably have involved parents who lived together in relatively small apartments, so that the mothers would have been strongly exposed to passive smoking during their pregnancies and the children will have been exposed subsequently. It is feasible that a passive smoking effect during pregnancy might have a deleterious effect on the subsequent susceptibility of the child, but this needs further study.

# References

Berkey, C. S., Ware, J. H., Dockery, D. W., Ferris, B. G., and Speizer, F. E. (1986). Indoor air pollution and pulmonary function growth in preadolescent children. *American Journal of Epidemiology,* **123,** 250–60.

Bisgaard, H., Dalgaard, P., and Nyboe, J. (1987). Risk factors for wheezing during infancy. *Acta Paediatrica Scandinavica,* **76,** 719–26.

Bland, M., Bewley, B. R., Pollard, V., and Banks, M. H. (1978). Effect of children's and parents' smoking on respiratory symptoms. *Archives of Diseases in Childhood,* **53,** 100–5.

Bonham, G. S. and Wilson, R. W. (1982). Minor error noted in study on child health in smokers' families. *American Journal of Public Health,* **72,** 403.

Butler, N. R. and Golding, J. (1986). *From birth to five. A study of the health and behaviour of Britain's five year olds.* Pergamon Press, Oxford.

Chamberlain, R., Chamberlain, G., Howlett, B., and Claireaux, A. (1975). *British Births 1970, vol I, The first week of life.* Heinemann, London.

Chamberlain, G., Phillip, E., Howlett, B., and Claireaux, A. (1978). *British Births 1970, vol II, Obstetric care.* Heinemann, London.

Chan, K. N., Elliman, A., Bryan, E. M., and Silverman, M. (1989a). Respiratory symptoms in children of low birthweight. *Archives of Diseases in Childhood,* **64,** 1294–304.

Chan, K. N., Noble-Jamieson, C. M., Elliman, A., Bryan, E. M., and Silverman, M. (1989b). Lung function in children of low birth weight. *Archives of Diseases in Childhood,* **64,** 1284–93.

Charlton, A. (1984). Children's coughs related to parental smoking. *British Medical Journal,* **288,** 1647–53.

Chen, Y. and Li, W-X. (1986). The effect of passive smoking on children's pulmonary function in Shanghai. *American Journal of Public Health,* **76,** 515–18.

Chen, Y., Li, W., and Yu, S. (1986). Influence of passive smoking on admissions for respiratory illness in early childhood. *British Medical Journal,* **293,** 303–6.

Clifford, R. D., Radford, M., Howell, J. B., and Holgate, S. T. (1989). Prevalence of respiratory symptoms among 7 and 11 year old schoolchildren and association with asthma. *Archives of Diseases in Childhood,* **64,** 1118–25.

Colley, J. R. T. (1974*a*). Respiratory symptoms in children and parental smoking and phlegm production. *British Medical Journal*, 2, 201–4.

Colley, J. R. T. (1974*b*). Influence of passive smoking and parental phlegm on pneumonia and bronchitis in early childhood. *Lancet*, ii, 1031–4.

Ekwo, E. E., Weinberger, M. M., Lachenbruch, P. A., and Huntley, W. H. (1983). Relationship of parental smoking and gas cooking to respiratory disease in children. *Chest*, 8, 662–8.

Fergusson, D. M., Horwood, L. J., and Shannon, F. T. (1980). Parental smoking and respiratory illness in infancy. *Archives of Diseases in Childhood*, 55, 358–61.

Fergusson, D. M., Horwood, L. J., Shannon, F. T., and Taylor, B. (1981). Parental smoking and lower respiratory illness in the first 3 years of life. *Journal of Epidemiology and Community Health*, 35, 180–4.

Fogelman, K. (1980). Smoking in pregnancy and subsequent development of the child. *Child: care, health and development*, 6, 233–49.

Gortmaker, S. L., Klein Walker, D., Jacobs, F. H., and Ruch-Ross, H. (1982). Parental smoking and risk of childhood asthma. *American Journal of Public Health*, 75, 574–9.

Harlap, S. and Davies, A. M. (1974). Infant admissions to hospital and maternal smoking. *Lancet*, i, 529–32.

Harrison, K. L. (1979). The effect of maternal smoking on neonatal leucocytes. *Australian and New Zealand Journal of Obstetrics and Gynaecology*, 19, 166–8.

Hosein, H. R., Corey, P., and Robertson, J. McD. (1989). The effect of domestic factors on respiratory symptoms and $FEV_1$. *International Journal of Epidemiology*, 18, 390–6.

Iversen, M., Birch, L., and Lundqvist, G. R. (1985). Middle ear infusion in children and the indoor environment: an epidemiological study. *Archives of Environmental Health*, 40, 74–9.

Lebowitz, M. D. and Burrows, B. (1976). Respiratory symptoms related to smoking habits of family adults. *Chest*, 69, 48–50.

Leeder, S. R., Corkhill, R. T., Irwig, L. M., Holland, W. W., and Colley, J. R. T. (1976*a*). Influence of family factors on the incidence of lower respiratory illness during the first year of life. *British Journal of Preventive and Social Medicine*, 30, 203–12.

Leeder, S. R., Corkhill, R. T., Irwig, L. M., Holland, W. W., and Colley, J. R. T. (1976*b*). Influence of family factors on asthma and wheezing during the first five years of life. *British Journal of Preventive and Social Medicine*, 30, 213–18.

Liard, R., Perdrizet, S., and Reinert, P. (1982). Wheezy bronchitis in infants and parents' smoking habits. *Lancet*, i, 334–5.

Lucas, A., Brooke, O. G., Cole, T. J., Morley, R., and Bamford, M. F. (1990). Food and drug reactions, wheezing and eczema in preterm infants. *Archives of Diseases in Childhood*, 65, 411–15.

Neuspiel, D. R., Rush, D., Butler, N. R., Golding, J., Bijur, P. E., and Kurzon, M. (1989). Parental smoking and post-infancy wheezing in children: a prospective cohort study. *American Journal of Public Health*, 79, 168–71.

Ogston, S. A., Florey, C. du V., and Walker, C. H. M. (1985). The Tayside infant morbidity and mortality study: effect on health of using gas for cooking. *British Medical Journal*, 290, 957–60.

Rantakallio, P. (1983). A follow-up study up to the age of 14 of children whose mothers smoked during pregnancy. *Acta Paediatrica Scandinavica*, 72, 747–53.

Said, G., Zalokar, J., Lellouch, J., and Patois, E. (1978). Parental smoking related to adenoidectomy and tonsillectomy in children. *Journal of Epidemiology and Community Health,* **32,** 97–101.

Schenker, M. B., Samet, J. M., and Speizer, F. E. (1983). Risk factors for childhood respiratory disease. The effect of host factors and home environmental exposures. *American Review of Respiratory Diseases,* **128,** 1038–43.

Tager, I. B., Weiss, S. T., Rosner, B., and Speizer, F. E. (1979). Effect of parental cigarette smoking on the pulmonary function of children. *American Journal of Epidemiology,* **110,** 15–26.

Tager, I. B., Weiss, S. T., Munoz, A., Rosner, B., and Speizer, F. E. (1983). Longitudinal study of the effects of maternal smoking on pulmonary function in children. *New England Journal of Medicine,* **309,** 699–702.

Taylor, B. and Wadsworth, J. (1987). Maternal smoking during pregnancy and lower respiratory tract illness in early life. *Archives of Diseases in Childhood,* **62,** 786–91.

Vogt, T. (1984). Effects of parental smoking on medical care utilization by children. *American Journal of Public Health,* **74,** 30–5.

Warren, C. P. W., Holmford-Strevens, V., Wang, C., *et al.* (1982). The relationship between smoking and total immunoglobulin E levels. *Journal of Allergies and Clinical Immunology,* **69,** 370–4.

Weiss, S. T., Tagner, I. B., Speizer, F. E., and Rosner, B. (1980). Persistent wheeze. Its relation to respiratory illness, cigarette smoking, and level of pulmonary function in a population sample of children. *American Reviews of Respiratory Disease,* **122,** 697–706.

# 11. Antenatal smoking, postnatal passive smoking, and the Sudden Infant Death Syndrome

*Jon Nicholl and Alicia O'Cathain*

## Introduction

Each year during the 1980s more than 6000 infants born in England and Wales died before reaching their first birthday. Roughly 20 per cent of all these infants deaths, 35 per cent of those occurring in the post-perinatal period, and 50 per cent of those occurring in the post-neonatal period, were certified as Sudden Infant Deaths ('cot' deaths) (Office of Population Censuses and Surveys 1987, 1988). The majority of these deaths are unexplained at necropsy (Arneil *et al.* 1985), and deaths are usually ascribed to the Sudden Infant Death Syndrome (SIDS) following Beckwith's (1970) definition.

In numerous epidemiological studies of SIDS, smoking—usually maternal smoking during pregnancy—has been one of the key associated characteristics. It has been claimed that: 'whenever data have been available for analysis it has been shown that infants of women who smoked during their pregnancy were at increased risk of sudden death in infancy' (Golding *et al.* 1985).

A review of the most recent literature available from several countries has shown this claim to be true, with only one exception in a study from Ireland (Matthews and O'Brien 1985).

Despite the strength and consistency of this evidence, doubt was cast on a recommendation in the report of the UK multicentre study of post-neonatal mortality (Knowelden *et al.* 1985) that Health Authorities should take action to reduce the prevalence of smoking during pregnancy and early infancy on the grounds that there was no evidence that this would affect the incidence of infant mortality or SIDS (Lancet 1985). The basis of this counterclaim was that the observed relationship between smoking and SIDS was merely a statistical association, and no causal link had been established. This in turn was interpreted as implying that reducing the prevalence of smoking would not necessarily reduce the incidence of SIDS.

It is possible that such doubts arise because those epidemiological studies that have looked at smoking have only studied maternal smoking during pregnancy, and have rarely attempted to be specific about which aspect of maternal smoking is important. Maternal smoking during pregnancy will usually be followed by postnatal smoking in the presence of the infant, and is often associated with smoking by the mother's partner. Little attempt has been made to ascertain whether the risk arises from the effects of antenatal smoking on the fetus or from the effects of postnatal exposure of infants to environmental tobacco smoke.

Most SIDS deaths are found to have some pathology at necropsy (Valdes-Dapena 1982; Knowelden *et al.* 1985) albeit insufficient to explain the death, and many have been found to have had some clinical evidence of disease before death (Stanton *et al.* 1978; Watson *et al.* 1981). The relevance of these findings remains debatable (Valman 1985), partly because such a wide variety of pathological and clinical evidence has been uncovered.

Some investigators looking at the epidemiology of SIDS have subdivided cases according to their age at death. Although the results of these studies have not always been consistent, some clear evidence of differences in the characteristics of older and younger SIDS cases has been reported. Thus Nicholl and O'Cathain (1989) found that the risk of SIDS occurring between 1 and 7 weeks of age rose sharply with an increase in the number of cigarettes per day smoked by their mothers during pregnancy. The risk of SIDS at older ages increased only slightly after adjustment for a variety of infant, maternal, and social factors.

As a result of these observations, and the identification of a specific cause in a few deaths otherwise indistinguishable from SIDS (Howat *et al.* 1985; Sonnabend *et al.* 1985), it is now widely believed that SIDS is not a single entity, and that a number of different causal mechanisms are involved. If this is the case then it is of course possible that different aspects of smoking may be important in different subgroups of SIDS deaths.

In this chapter an attempt is made to unravel the roles of maternal smoking during pregnancy and postnatal passive smoking in SIDS deaths, using data from the UK multicentre study (Knowelden *et al.* 1985) to make the evidence of an association more specific and to examine the causal hypothesis in the light of this evidence.

## Methods

Data on 988 babies who died at between the ages of 1 week and 2 years and 773 controls matched for date and place of birth were collected for the UK multicentre study of post-neonatal mortality. Details of the data and methods have been described previously (Knowelden *et al.* 1985). Eight centres were included in the study, which ran between 1976 and 1979, and data were obtained on each death from hospital records, home interviews, general practitioner and health visitor records, and necropsy findings. At the home interview questions were asked about how many cigarettes per day the mother smoked during pregnancy and about how many cigarettes the husband/consort usually smokes per day.

Excluding babies who did not have a thorough necropsy, there were 303 babies in the study (31 per cent of the total) whose deaths were not explained or expected, and who would usually be labelled SIDS, in accordance with the definition of Beckwith (1970). These are the subject of this account. Nearly half (42 per cent) of these babies were completely symptomless before death, one-fifth (21 per cent) had non-specific symptoms and the remainder had symptoms of specific illnesses (typically of upper respiratory tract infections) not sufficient to explain the deaths. For these 303 SIDS cases there were 277 matched controls.

For comparison with the results of other studies, estimates have been made of the overall risk of SIDS associated with mothers who smoked during pregnancy, irrespective of their partner's smoking habits, using the ratio of the odds for the cases and controls. This estimated relative risk has also been adjusted to take account of birthweight, maternal age and gravidity, and the state of the family's housing.

The risk of SIDS associated with maternal smoking has been estimated independently of the risk associated with partner's smoking, and vice versa, by fitting logistic regression models to the data (Breslow and Day 1980). The resulting estimated relative risk associated with maternal smoking has also been adjusted for birth weight. These estimates for the risk of SIDS associated independently with maternal and partner's smoking have been calculated separately for four groups of SIDS cases with different ages of death (1–7, 8–15, 16–23, and 24+ weeks).

# Results

The smoking habits of both the mother and her partner were known for 242 of the 303 SIDS cases in the multicentre data and for 251 of the 277 matched controls (Table 11.1). The overall estimated relative risk of SIDS in the infants of mothers who smoked during pregnancy, whether or not their partners smoked, based on the odds ratio, was 2.42 (95 per cent confidence interval (CI) 1.67, 3.50).

Adjustment for birth weight using four birth weight groups (< 2500 g, 2500–2999 g, 3000–3499 g, and $\geq 3500$ g) reduced the estimated risk only marginally to 2.18 (95 per cent CI 1.47, 3.22). Adjustment for maternal age, gravidity, and housing repair together also reduced the estimated risk by a small amount to 1.87 (95 per cent CI 1.27, 2.76).

When a logistic regression model was fitted to the data in Table 11.1 there was no evidence of any interaction in the effect of maternal and partner's smoking ($\chi^2 = 0.97$; df = 1; $P > 0.3$). The resulting estimate of the independent risk of maternal smoking was 2.13 (95 per cent CI 1.45, 3.13), and of the independent risk associated with the partner's smoking was 1.63 (95 per cent CI 1.11, 2.40). Excluding the four cases whose birth weights were not recorded, the independent maternal smoking risk estimate was 2.21 and this fell

**Table 11.1** Estimated risk of SIDS associated with families' smoking status relative to the risk in non-smoking families

| Smoking status | No. of cases | No. of controls | Crude odds ratio | Estimated* relative risk (95% confidence interval) |
|---|---|---|---|---|
| Mother didn't smoke in pregnancy. Partner doesn't smoke | 54 | 97 | — | — |
| Mother didn't smoke in pregnancy. Partner smokes | 52 | 67 | 1.39 | 1.63 (1.11, 2.40) |
| Mother smoked during pregnancy. Partner doesn't smoke | 30 | 32 | 1.68 | 2.13 (1.45, 3.13) |
| Mother smoked during pregnancy. Partner smokes | 106 | 55 | 3.46 | — |
| All (known) | 242 | 251 | — | — |

* Independent risks associated with maternal and partner's smoking estimated from the multiple logistic regression model.

to 1.98 (95 per cent CI 1.32, 2.96) after adjustment for birth weight. A similar analysis of the independent risk associated with maternal and partner's smoking in each of the four age-at-death groups found that the estimated risk in the infants of mothers who smoked, relative to that in the infants of mothers who did not smoke, fell from 3.98 in young babies (< 8 weeks old), to 1.41 in older babies (over 24 weeks) (Fig. 11.1). The estimated risk associated with partner's smoking, however, showed the opposite effect and increased from 1.49 in the youngest babies to 2.62 in the oldest group.

## Discussion

### Antenatal and postnatal smoking

As maternal smoking during pregnancy will usually be followed by postnatal smoking, the risk of SIDS associated with maternal antenatal smoking as usually estimated actually represents the risk associated with either antenatal smoking or postnatal smoking or both. On the other hand, smoking by the mother's partner is only likely to increase the risk of SIDS as a result of the consequent postnatal passive smoking of the infant. Consequently, the finding we have presented here—that there is a significant and independent

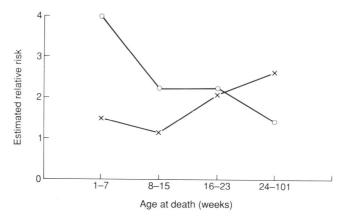

**Fig. 11.1.** Estimated relative risk of SIDS at different ages due to the independent effects of mother's smoking (o) and her partner's smoking (x).

increase in the risk of SIDS associated with the partner's smoking—strongly suggests that postnatal passive smoking does play a role in the risk of SIDS.

The finding of an increased risk with the partner's smoking is in accordance with results presented by Cameron and Williams (1986) who found that 'father smokes' was a very highly significant risk factor for SIDS and included it in a birth scoring system to identify infants at risk of SIDS. In contrast, Bergman and Wiesner (1976) found no association with 'paternal smoking', but their evidence was based on a response rate of only 56 per cent to a mailed questionnaire to 100 parents.

The finding that the risk of SIDS is related to passive postnatal smoking raises the question of whether any part of the frequently identified risk associated with the maternal smoking during pregnancy is due to antenatal maternal smoking, or whether this risk is entirely due to the postnatal smoking that almost invariably follows antenatal smoking. The estimated relative risk associated independently with maternal smoking (2.13) was greater than that independently associated with the partner's smoking (1.63) and this suggests that both antenatal and postnatal passive smoking may increase the risk. Further evidence for this comes from finding that the relative risk associated with maternal smoking is very large in the neonatal period and immediately afterwards ($RR = 4.0$) but thereafter falls to a level similar to that for the risk associated with the partner's smoking. Moreover, the risk associated with the partner's smoking increases with the infant's age and is most marked over the age of 15 weeks. These results provide some evidence that there is an increased risk associated with *both* maternal smoking during pregnancy *per se* and postnatal passive smoking by the infant.

Considering first the risk associated with antenatal maternal smoking, it is well known both that this affects birth weight adversely and that low birth weight is associated with an increased risk of SIDS. Adjusting the estimated risk associated with maternal smoking independent of partner's smoking for birth weight reduces it from 2.2 to 2.0, and this is in line with results from other studies that have done this. It is not surprising that the risk does not disappear altogether because of the postnatal passive smoking component. On the other hand, the risk associated with maternal smoking adjusted for birth weight, which has been found in the present and other studies is at a level similar to that associated with the partner's smoking. As the latter risk will be due almost entirely to postnatal passive smoking, the antenatal component of the risk associated with maternal smoking may be due only to the effect on birth weight.

With regard to the risk associated with postnatal passive smoking, it is well known both that postnatal passive smoking leads to more infant and childhood morbidity, especially from lower respiratory tract illness (Colley *et al.* 1974; Leader *et al.* 1976; Fergusson *et al.* 1980; Yue Chen *et al.* 1986; Evans and Golding Chapter 10), and that SIDS cases commonly have clinical and pathological evidence of respiratory disease (Stanton *et al.* 1978; Knowelden *et al.* 1985). Unfortunately, it is not clear whether there is any connection between these terminal diseases and the subsequent infant deaths. It may be the case that smoking causes respiratory infections unrelated to the occurrence of SIDs, but also has some other unknown effect, which does contribute to the occurrence of SIDS. Peterson (1981), as well as agreeing that maternal smoking probably acts both through an effect on intra-uterine growth and as a result of postnatal passive smoking, has postulated that the postnatal effects could also be due to inhibition of postnatal development.

## Does smoking cause SIDS?

As Hume pointed out 250 years ago, all 'causes' are merely associations with particular qualities (Hume 1970). In the absence of experimental evidence, which is regarded by many as a necessary and sufficient condition for identifying causal associations, epidemiologists have identified a number of criteria (Elwood 1988) that, taken together, would make it: 'more provident to act on the basis that the association is causal rather than to await further evidence' (McMahon and Pugh 1970).

The most important criteria are strength and consistency between studies. Table 11.2 presents results from 11 studies in seven countries relating to the association of maternal smoking during pregnancy and SIDS. These studies are all those published during the 1980s that included an estimate of the relative risk associated with maternal smoking, or data from which the risk could be calculated. In addition, Steele and Langworth's original 1966 study is included, as is Bergman and Wiesner's 1976 study of passive smoking, which is the only other study to have addressed this issue. With only two exceptions, these 11 studies show that the risk to infants whose mothers smoked during pregnancy was between two and three times that for infants whose mothers

**Table 11.2** The association of maternal smoking during pregnancy and SIDS. Summary of results from recent major reports from several countries

| Authors | Date of publication | District, | Country | Unadjusted odds of SIDS for smokers | (95% CI) | Social factors taken into account | Adjusted odds | Odds adjusted for birthweight | Dose–response relationship |
|---|---|---|---|---|---|---|---|---|---|
| Present study | | 8 centres, | England | 2.4 | (1.7, 3.5) | Maternal age, parity, housing conditions | 1.9 | 2.2 | Yes |
| Gilbert et al. | 1990 | Avon, | England | 2.4* | (1.5, 4.1) | | | | |
| Haglund and Cnattingius | 1990 | | Sweden | 2.3† | (1.6, 3.0) | Maternal age, parity | 2.1‡ | 2.0‡ | Yes |
| Kraus et al. | 1989 | | USA | 2.0‡ | (1.2, 3.0) | | | 1.8‡ | |
| Malloy et al. | 1988 | Missouri, | USA | 2.9 | (2.4, 3.6) | Mother's marital status, education level, age, and parity | 1.9 | 1.8§ | Yes |

| Author | Year | Location | Relative risk | (95% CI) | Other risk factors considered | | |
|---|---|---|---|---|---|---|---|
| Rintahaka and Hirvonen | 1986 | Finland | 4.1 | (2.4, 7.1) | Reported as 'most significant risk factor independent from other risk factors' | | |
| Cameron and Williams | 1986 | Melbourne, Australia | 2.7 | (1.9, 3.8) | Unemployment, housing, parents' age | Significant but not given | Significant but not given |
| Matthews and O'Brien | 1985 | Dublin, Ireland | 0.7 | (0.3, 1.9) | | | |
| Murphy et al. | 1982 | Cardiff, Wales | 2.8† | (1.6, 4.0) | | | |
| Bergman and Wiesner | 1976 | Seattle, USA | 2.2 | (1.1, 4.3) | Maternal education | 2.1‖ | Yes |
| Steele and Langworth | 1966 | Ontario, Canada | 2.5 | (1.4, 4.4) | | 1.5¶ | Yes |

\* Sudden unexpected deaths.

† Relative risk estimated from a prospective study.

‡ Estimated from those reported for varying levels of cigarette consumption.

§ Adjusted for both social factors and birth weight.

‖ Adjusted risk associated with reported post-natal maternal smoking.

¶ Odds of SIDS in babies weighing < 2500 g.

did not smoke. Only the Irish study found a lower and non-significant risk, whilst the study from Finland estimated the relative risk to be greater than 4.0. In all cases, when these odds have been adjusted for birth weight, they have been diminished to between 1.5 and 2.0, but have remained statistically significant. Adjusting for various social factors, such as mother's age, education, and marital status, has also reduced the estimated odds to about 2.0 but, again, these adjusted odds have usually been found to be significant.

The next most important criteria are coherence with other known facts and biological plausibility. It was suggested earlier that the risk associated with maternal smoking during pregnancy has both an antenatal and a postnatal component. Many other studies have shown that cigarette smoking in pregnancy retards fetal development and the finding of an increased risk, particularly in young babies under 8 weeks old, associated with maternal antenatal smoking is entirely coherent with this. With regard to postnatal passive smoking, the suggestion of its possibly causal role is coherent with the theories that ascribe SIDS to congenital respiratory abnormalities (Wiel 1980; Milner 1987), or to respiratory infections (Franciosi 1985). This has been reported to be the case particularly in older infants (Williams *et al.* 1984), where the present study found the risk associated with passive smoking to be the greatest. These findings would all support the hypothesis that smoking may be a contributory cause of SIDS, and that reducing the prevalence of smoking would reduce the incidence of SIDS. There could, also, be a direct link between smoking and SIDS if the risk were related to the action of a toxic agent in tobacco smoke such as carbon monoxide (Watkins and Strope 1986).

Another criterion for establishing causality, mentioned by Bradford Hill (1965), is that there should be a dose–response relationship between the supposed causal agent and the disease in question. As Table 11.2 shows, all five studies that have looked for such a relationship found an increase in risk with the number of cigarettes smoked daily.

Taken together, the evidence of strength, consistency, plausibility, and the dose–response relationship argue strongly that smoking should be considered to be causally related to SIDS. If, however, it is still felt that a causal relationship should never be assumed until Bradford Hill's last criterion of experimental evidence is satisfied, then perhaps serious consideration should be given to developing and testing a population intervention programme that, amongst other things, should attempt to reduce the prevalence of both antenatal and postnatal smoking in an experimental population.

It has been estimated that if maternal smoking could be eliminated altogether then the overall infant death rate could be reduced by 10 per cent (Malloy *et al.* 1988) and the SIDS death rate by 27 per cent (Haglund and Cnattingius 1990). With more than 1000 babies dying each year in England and Wales from causes ascribed to SIDS these estimates suggest that the deaths of many infants in the first weeks of their lives might be prevented. With such large rewards, and such strong evidence that they might be achiev-

able, at least in part, it would seem reasonable now to expect explicit programmes and action by Health Authorities to implement the recommendations
of the multicentre report—especially as evidence is mounting that the rate of
decline in smoking amongst young women is slowing down.

## Acknowledgements

The secondary analysis of the multicentre data was supported by the Foundation for the Study of Infant Deaths. The original study and analysis was
funded by the DoH, who, together with Trent Regional Health Authority,
maintain the Medical Care Research Unit. We are grateful for their support.

## References

Arneil, G. C., Brooke, H., Gibson, A. A. M., Horvie, A., McIntosh, H., and Patrick,
    W. S. A. (1985). National post-perinatal infant mortality and cot death study,
    Scotland 1981–1982. *Lancet*, **i**, 740–3.
Beckwith, J. B. (1970). Observations on the pathological anatomy of the sudden
    infant death syndrome. In *Sudden infant death syndrome*, (Proceedings of the 2nd
    international conference on the causes of sudden death in infants), (ed. A. B. Berg-
    man, J. B. Beckwith, and C. G. Ray), p. 83. University of Washington Press,
    Seattle.
Bergman, A. B. and Wiesner, B. A. (1976). Relationship of passive cigarette-smoking
    to Sudden Infant Death Syndrome. *Paediatrics*, **58(5)**, 665–8.
Bradford Hill, A. B. (1965). *The environment and disease: Association or causation?*
    Proceedings of the Royal Society of Medicine (Section of Occupational Medicine),
    **58(1)**, pp. 295–300. January 14th.
Breslow, N. E. and Day, N. E. (1980). *Statistical methods in cancer research, vol. 1,
    The analysis of case-control studies*. IARC Scientific Publications No. 32, Lyon.
Cameron, M. H. and Williams, A. L. (1986). Development and testing of scoring
    systems for predicting infants with high-risk of Sudden Infant Death Syndrome in
    Melbourne. *Australian Paediatric Journal*, (Suppl.), 37–45.
Colley, J. R. T., Holland, W. W., and Corkhill, R. T. (1974). The influence of passive
    smoking and parental phlegm on pneumonia and bronchitis in early childhood.
    *Lancet*, **ii**, 1031–4.
Elwood, M. J. (1988). *Causal relationships in medicine. A practical system for critical
    appraisal*. Oxford University Press, Oxford.
Fergusson, D. M., Horwood, L. J., and Shannon, F. T. (1980). Parental smoking and
    respiratory illness in infancy. *Archives of Diseases of Childhood*, **55**, 358–61.
Franciosi, R. A. (1985). Respiratory infections as a trigger for Sudden Infant Death
    Syndrome. *Minnesota Medicine*, **April 1985**, 271–2.
Gilbert, R. E., Fleming, P. J., Azaz, Y., and Rudd, P. (1990). Signs of illness
    preceding sudden unexpected death in infants. *British Medical Journal*, **300**, 1237–9.
Golding, J., Limerick, S., and McFarlane, A. (1985). *Sudden infant death. Patterns
    puzzles and problems*, p. 56. Open Books, Taunton.
Haglund, B. and Cnattingius, S. (1990). Cigarette smoking as a risk factor for Sudden
    Infant Death Syndrome: A population-based study. *American Journal of Public
    Health*, **80(1)**, 29–32.

Howat, A. J., Bennett, M. K., Variend, S., Shaw, L., and Engel, P. C. (1985). Defects of metabolism of fatty acids in the sudden infant death syndrome. *British Medical Journal*, **290**, 1771–3.

Hume, D. (1970). *A treatise of human nature. Book I* (ed. D. G. C. Macnabb), (3rd impression), pp. 180–93. Fontana, London.

Knowelden, J., Keeling, J., and Nicholl, J. (1985). *A multicentre study of post-neonatal mortality*. HMSO, London.

Kraus, J. P., Greenland, S., and Bulterys, M. (1989). Risk factors for Sudden Infant Death Syndrome in the US collaborative perinatal project. *International Journal of Epidemiology*, **18(1)**, 113–20.

Lancet (1985). Post-neonatal mortality in the UK. *Lancet*, **i**, 322.

Leader, S. R., Corkhill, R., Irwig, L. M., Holland, W. W., and Colley, J. R. T. (1976). Influence of family factors on the incidence of lower respiratory illness during the first year of life. *British Journal of Preventive and Social Medicine*, **30**, 203–12.

Malloy, M. H., Kleinman, J. C., Land, G. H., and Schramm, W. F. (1988). The association of maternal smoking with age and cause of infant deaths. *American Journal of Epidemiology*, **128(1)**, 46–55.

Matthews, T. G. and O'Brien, S. J. (1985). Perinatal epidemiological characteristics of the Sudden Infant Death Syndrome in an Irish population. *Irish Medical Journal*, **78**, 251–3.

McMahon, B. and Pugh, T. G. (1970). *Epidemiology, principles and methods*. Brown and Co., Boston.

Milner, A. D. (1987). Recent theories on the cause of cot death. *British Medical Journal*, **295**, 1366–8.

Murphy, J. F., Newcombe, R. G., and Sibert, J. R. (1982). The epidemiology of sudden infant death syndrome. *Journal of Epidemiology and Community Health*, **36**, 17–21.

Nicholl, J. P. and O'Cathain, A. (1989). Epidemiology of babies dying at different ages from the sudden infant death syndrome. *Journal of Epidemiology and Community Health*, **43(2)**, 133–9.

Office of Population Censuses and Surveys (OPCS) (1987). *Mortality statistics, childhood 1985*, Series DH3, No. 19. HMSO, London.

Office of Population Censuses and Surveys (OPCS) (1988). Sudden Infant Deaths 1985–87. *OPCS Monitor*, DH3 88/3. Government Statistical Service, London.

Peterson, D. R. (1981). The sudden infant death syndrome—reassessment of growth retardation in relation to maternal smoking and the hypoxia hypothesis. *American Journal of Epidemiology*, **113(5)**, 583–9.

Rintahaka, P. J. and Hirvonen, J. (1986). The epidemiology of sudden infant death syndrome in Finland in 1969–1980. *Forensic Science International*, **30**, 219–33.

Sonnabend, O. A. R., Sonnabend, W. F. F., Krech, H., Molz, G., and Sigrist, J. (1985). Continuous microbiological and pathological study of 70 sudden and unexpected infant deaths. Toxigenic intestinal *Clostridium botulinum* infection in 9 cases of sudden infant death syndrome. *Lancet*, **i**, 237–41.

Stanton, A. N., Downham, M. A. P. S., and Oakley, J. R. (1978). Controlled study of terminal symptoms and the action taken for them in the first 100 sudden unexpected home deaths in the DHSS multicentre study of post-neonatal deaths. *Archives of Diseases in Childhood*, **53**, 834–5.

Steele, R. and Langworth, J. T. (1966). The relationship of antenatal and postnatal factors to sudden unexpected death in infancy. *Canadian Medical Association Journal*, **94**, 1165–71.

Valdes-Dapena, M. (1982). The pathologist and the sudden infant death syndrome. *American Journal of Pathology,* **106(1),** 118–31.

Valman, B. (1985). Preventing infant deaths (editorial). *British Medical Journal,* **290,** 339–40.

Watkins, C. G. and Strope, G. L. (1986). Chronic carbon monoxide poisoning as a major constituting factor in the sudden infant death syndrome. *American Journal of Diseases in Childhood,* **140,** 619.

Watson, E., Gardner, A., and Carpenter, R. G. (1981). An epidemiological and sociological study of unexpected deaths in infancy in nine areas of southern England: II symptoms and patterns of care. *Medicine, Science and Law,* **21,** 89–98.

Wiel, J. V. (1980). Familial factors, ventilatory control, and sudden infant death. *New England Journal of Medicine,* **302(9),** 517–19.

Williams, A. L., Uren, E. C., and Bretherton, L. (1984). Respiratory viruses and sudden infant death. *British Medical Journal,* **288,** 1491–3.

Yue Chen, Wanxian Li, Shunzhang Yu (1986). Influence of passive smoking on admissions for respiratory illness in early childhood. *British Medical Journal,* **293,** 303–6.

# 12. Exposure to passive cigarette smoking and child development: an updated critical review

*David Rush*

## Introduction

While maternal cigarette smoking during pregnancy is closely related to the growth and survival of the fetus (Rush and Kass 1972), the nature and extent of effects on later development of the child are not clearly understood. In an attempt to clarify current knowledge, this review (an update of Rush and Callahan 1989) describes the design and some of the strengths and weaknesses of each of the studies known, and then summarizes, across studies, relationships with somatic, cognitive, and behavioural development.

## Possible confounding factors

The major problem of drawing inference from observational studies comparing developmental outcomes of offspring of smokers and non-smokers is a failure to allow fully for social differences, which strongly influence both the smoking habit and a variety of social and behavioural factors. However, caution should be taken in assuming that it is possible to match or statistically control for them. Smokers are known to differ in behaviour, personality, and social status from non-smokers (Heath 1958; Lilienfeld 1959; Harrison and Kass 1967; Reiter 1970; Schneider and Houston 1970) and such factors are strongly related to child development. While it is necessary to control for such differences in analysis it is almost surely illusory to assume that it can be done fully. Certainly, in northern Europe and the English-speaking countries, smokers are, on average, very likely to still be at a disadvantage, even after stratifying on any social class index, such as occupational status.

Precisely this effect was observed by Rantakallio (1983) in her study of child development at age 14 in northern Finland. Children whose mothers had smoked during pregnancy were compared with children matched on mother's marital status, age, parity, and place of residence. She found that, with minor exceptions:

> Within each social class of the husband, the smoking mother was in a less favourable position (in terms of unemployment, sick leave or sick pension, not living with the family, or having died) than her non-smoking counterpart . . .

Thus, within social class strata, smoking was associated with consistently adverse conditions for child development.

In spite of such likely confounding, differences in cognitive and neurological development in childhood reported in many studies to be associated with parental smoking were only minimally controlled for social factors, and while they may have been highly significant statistically, they cannot be straightforwardly interpreted as having been caused by smoking.

## Review of specific studies

### The National Child Development Study (NCDS)

All 16 000 children born in one week in March 1958 in Great Britain were studied at birth, and at ages seven, 11, and 16 (Butler and Bonham 1963; Butler and Alberman 1969; Davie *et al.* 1972; Butler and Goldstein 1973; Fogelman 1980). Measures of physical, behavioural, and cognitive development have been reported from each postnatal follow-up, and those that were related to maternal smoking in pregnancy are presented in Table 12.1.

Definitions of smoking and data analytic procedures varied somewhat at different ages (see footnotes to Table 12.1). Raw differences were adjusted for social class and several other pertinent factors for all four outcomes reported at age 11, and for parental height at age seven. For reading and social adjustment at age seven, and for all measures at age 16, the reported results were adjusted for birth weight. Adjusting for birth weight tends systematically to underestimate the relationship of smoking during pregnancy with later child development, as cigarette smoking in pregnancy causes lowered birth weight. The reported decrements in reading achievement at age seven that were controlled for birth weight, 1.0 months in children of light smokers (< 10 cigarettes/day) and 3.9 months in children of heavy smokers (10+ cigarettes/day) were thus likely to be underestimates of real relationships.

At age seven much, but not the greatest part, of the relationship between maternal smoking during pregnancy with depressed stature was associated with lowered birth weight: among 7-year-old children of lighter smokers, the height difference was reduced from 0.60 cm to 0.40 cm by controlling for birth weight, and among children of heavy smokers, from 0.99 cm to 0.65 cm.

At age 11, with adjustment for social class, children of lighter smokers were shorter by 0.57 cm, retarded by 4.5 months in general ability, 3.1 months in reading achievement, and 4.7 months in mathematics achievement, compared to children of non-smokers. For children of heavier smokers, the respective differences were 1.0 cm, 3.6 months, 3.1 months, and 4.9 months, compared to children of non-smokers. These differences were all highly significant. Controlling for paternal occupational status as well as the child's sex, maternal age, parity, and the number of younger sibs caused an average reduction in

**Table 12.1** Differences in ability and achievement (in months, except as noted) and in height (cm): smokers versus non-smokers

| | Cigarettes/day from fourth month of gestation | | | | | |
| --- | --- | --- | --- | --- | --- | --- |
| | <10 | | | 10+ | | |
| Age (years) | Unadjusted | (1) | (2) | Unadjusted | (1) | (2) |
| **General ability** | | | | | | |
| 11 | −8.0*** | −4.5*** | — | −8.0*** | −3.6*** | — |
| **Reading** | | | | | | |
| 7 | — | — | −1.0*** | — | — | −3.9*** |
| 11 | −7.4*** | −3.1*** | — | −9.0*** | −3.1*** | — |
| 16 | — | — | −0.087***[1] | — | — | −0.117***[1] |
| **Mathematics** | | | | | | |
| 11 | −7.1*** | −4.7*** | — | −8.5*** | −4.9*** | — |
| 16 | — | — | −0.14***[1] | — | — | −0.18***[1] |
| **Height** | | | | | | |
| 7 | −0.9[2] | −0.60[2] | −0.40[2] | −1.3[2] | −0.99[2] | −0.65[2] |
| 11 | −0.95*** | −0.57*** | — | −1.6*** | −1.0*** | — |
| 16[3] | — | — | −0.57* | — | — | −0.89* |
| Boys | | | | | | |
| Girls | — | — | 0.19 | — | — | −0.39 |

(1) adjusted for age (except at 16), sex, maternal height and parity, paternal occupational status, and n younger sibs.
(2) as (1), plus gestation and birth weight.
[1] SD units (age not included in regression: cannot be translated into months).
[2] Statistical tests not presented.
[3] Smoking categories: 10 cigs/day; > 10 cigs/day.
* $P < 0.05$; ** $P < 0.01$; *** $P < 0.001$.
From The National Child Development Study (Great Britain: 1958 Births).
Authors: Davie *et al.* (1972) at seven years of age; Butler and Goldstein (1973) at eleven years of age; Fogelman (1980) at sixteen years of age.

the association of prenatal smoking with the same four outcomes of 48 per cent. At age 16, only results adjusted for birth weight were presented. Effects on height were greater among boys but, overall, differences appeared to be relatively stable over time.

## National Collaborative Perinatal Project (NCPP)

The NCPP followed 58 000 pregnancies at 12 US teaching centres, starting in the late 1950s, and most of the surviving children were then periodically examined to age seven. Six publications are known that related maternal smoking to later child development, all but one (Broman *et al.* 1975) looking at the effect of smoking in pregnancy.

Garn *et al.* (1980, 1981) found increased rates of low neonatal Apgar scores and low Bayley motor and mental scores at 1 year of age among both white and black babies, where the mothers had been heavy smokers in pregnancy (Table 12.2). The only impressive adverse association was among infants of the few women who smoked over 40 cigarettes a day (96 whites and 24 blacks, and somewhat fewer children at 1 year of age). Other smaller studies have not been able to replicate these findings (see below). Social and other differences between smokers and non-smokers were not controlled, and no statistical tests were presented.

**Table 12.2** Low Apgar scores at birth and low Bayley scores at 8 months—maternal smoking in pregnancy

|  | Cigarettes/day in pregnancy | | | |
|---|---|---|---|---|
|  | 0 | <21 | 21–40 | 41+ |
| % Apgar score < 5 | | | | |
| One minute | | | | |
|   whites | 12.8 | 14.0 | 13.7 | 20.8 |
|   blacks | 12.0 | 13.7 | 14.2 | 31.8 |
| Five minutes | | | | |
|   whites | 2.2 | 2.9 | 3.1 | 3.3 |
|   blacks | 3.5 | 4.0 | 7.2 | 12.5 |
| % Bayley scores < 26 (motor) and < 74 (mental) at 8 months | | | | |
| Whites | | | | |
|   motor | 10.1 | 10.2 | 13.8 | 15.8 |
|   mental | 10.2 | 10.5 | 12.5 | 15.8 |
| Blacks | | | | |
|   motor | 9.7 | 10.2 | 11.8 | 11.8 |
|   mental | 15.2 | 15.2 | 17.9 | 23.5 |

From Garn *et al.* (1980, 1981). The National Collaborative Perinatal Project (NCPP). 58000 pregnancies at 12 teaching centres, born in the late 1950s and followed to age seven. This table is based on 43492 live-born singletons.

Hardy and Mellits (1972) performed a well-controlled small study among the Baltimore subsample of the NCPP. They matched 88 infants of women who smoked 10 or more cigarettes a day during pregnancy for race, sex, date of delivery, maternal age, and years of schooling, with 88 control subjects; and for 55 they selected a second control subject also matched for birth weight (Table 12.3). As numbers were small, power was low and few differences could be expected to be significant. At age seven, children of smokers

**Table 12.3** Differences between weight, length, and head circumference between infants in mothers who smoked 10 or more cigarettes/day in pregnancy and infants of non-smokers

| Age | 88 controls[1] | | | 55 controls[2] | | |
|---|---|---|---|---|---|---|
| | Weight (g) | Length (cm) | Head circ. (cm) | Weight (g) | Length (cm) | Head circ. (cm) |
| Birth | −250*** | −1.34*** | −0.32 | −20 | −0.26 | 0.01 |
| 1 year | −250 | −0.13* | −0.36 | 170 | 0.32 | −0.19 |
| 4 years | −110 | −0.70 | −0.39* | 0 | 0.15 | −0.14 |
| 7 years | −650 | −1.00 | −0.17 | −400 | 0.62 | −0.07 |

* $P < 0.05$; *** $P < 0.001$.
From Hardy and Mellits (1972). Subjects were 88 infants of women registered in the Baltimore subsample of NCPP. Controls were:
[1] 88 infants of non-smokers matched for race, sex, date of delivery, maternal age, and schooling and
[2] 55 infants also matched for birth weight.

were 1 cm shorter than the children of mothers who had not smoked, but not shorter than the birth-weight-matched controls: later somatic differences in stature thus appeared to be mediated by prenatal growth retardation. Among cognitive measures, only the spelling scale of the Wide Range Achievement Test (WRAT) was significantly depressed (Table 12.4). However, performance by subjects was worse than controls on all subtests.

Broman *et al.* (1975) found a small (1-point) but significant advantage in IQ at age four among white children whose mothers had never smoked, compared to those whose mothers had smoked (Table 12.5), and a small but highly significant *advantage* for infants of black smokers compared to infants of black non-smokers (1.1 points); social differences were not controlled.

Nichols and Chen (1981) performed an elaborate investigation of minimal brain damage among 30 000 NCPP children examined at age seven. Maternal smoking during pregnancy was strongly and significantly related to all three components of minimal brain damage—learning difficulties, hyperactivity–impulsivity, and neurological soft signs. Table 12.6 shows children of women smoking 20 or more cigarettes a day during pregnancy were 25 per cent more likely to have learning difficulties, 28 per cent more likely to show hyperactivity–impulsivity behaviour, and 15 per cent more likely to have soft signs. In each case the association was stronger where the problems were severe. These results were not controlled for social differences between smokers and non-smokers.

Among 140 full-term white sibling pairs studied by Naeye (1981) in which the mother smoked in only one of her pregnancies, the children exposed to

**Table 12.4** Differences between mean Apgar score and developmental tests between infants in mothers who smoked 10 or more cigarettes/day in pregnancy and infants of non-smokers

|  | 88 controls[1] | 55 controls[2] |
|---|---|---|
| Mean Apgar score |  |  |
| Lowest | 0.47 | 0.70 |
| 5 minutes | −0.11 | −0.11 |
| Neurologically abnormal | 6% (10% versus 4%) | 4% (10% versus 6%) |
| IQ, 4 years | −1.20 | −0.10 |
| IQ, 7 years | −1.35 | −1.49 |
| WRAT at age 7 |  |  |
| Spelling | −2.62* | −2.16 |
| Reading | −1.86 | −2.36 |
| Maths | 0.89 | −0.37 |
| Bender Gestalt | −0.24 | −0.67 |
| Draw a person | −2.91 | 2.47 |
| ITPA | −0.09 | 0.69 |

\* $P < 0.05$

From Hardy and Mellits (1972). Subjects were 88 infants of women registered in the Baltimore subsample of NCPP. Controls were:

[1] 88 infants of non-smokers matched for race, sex, date of delivery, maternal age, and schooling and

[2] 55 infants also matched for birth weight.

**Table 12.5** Mean IQ in 4-year-olds classified whether mothers had ever smoked up to the time of birth

|  | Mean IQ | |
|---|---|---|
|  | Mothers never smoked | Mothers had smoked |
| White | 105.3 | 104.3** |
| Black | 90.8 | 91.9*** |

\*\* $P < 0.01$; \*\*\* $P < 0.001$.

Statistical tests used not specified. No adjustment was made for any social or other differences between smokers and non-smokers.

From Broman *et al.* (1975) 4-year-old children from NCPP classified by whether mothers had *ever* smoked, to time of birth.

**Table 12.6** Relative risk of problems in children whose mothers smoked 20+ cigarettes/day during pregnancy, versus children of non-smokers

| Cigarettes/day | Learning difficulties | | Hyperactivity | | Soft signs (NS) |
|---|---|---|---|---|---|
| | All | Severe | All | Severe | |
| 20+ | 1.25*** | 1.44*** | 1.28*** | 1.32*** | 1.15** |
| 40+ | 1.46** | 1.66* | 1.54** | 1.63* | 1.34* |

\* $P < 0.05$; \*\* $P < 0.01$; \*\*\* $P < 0.001$.
   Statistical analysis: on discriminant analysis, among pregnancy and delivery factors, number of cigarettes/day was significantly related to learning difficulties (third strongest discriminator), severe learning difficulties (second strongest), hyperactivity (strongest), severe hyperactivity (strongest), soft signs (strongest), severe 'soft signs' (rank order not given).
   From Nichols and Chen (1981) 7-year-old children.

cigarette smoke were 1.7 cm shorter at age seven than their sibs where the mother had not smoked ($P < 0.001$). Among white term children, those of 1634 light smokers during pregnancy (< 20 cigarettes/day) were 1.1 cm shorter at age seven, and of 1231 heavy smokers (20+ cigarettes/day) 2.1 cm shorter, than children of 1632 non-smokers (calculated from the author's data). All differences were highly significant. However, sex, birth order, and social differences were not controlled in the sibling study, nor was there any explanation why blacks (who comprised nearly half the study population) were not included in analysis.

   Naeye and Peters (1984) reported on some aspects of the mental development and maternal smoking of 482 7-year-olds from the Boston Lying-In Hospital subpopulation of the NCPP (Table 12.7), a subset of 2903 white children from the middle socio-economic status group (Table 12.8), and among 578 same-sex sibling pairs, balanced for birth order, in which the mother smoked in only one pregnancy, presumably from all NCPP sites (Table 12.9).

   Among the Boston Lying-In Hospital population there were significant decrements in spelling and reading (but not arithmetic) scales on the WRAT in a regression analysis adjusted for several possible confounding factors. Children of smokers were rated as significantly less attentive and more active on a five-point scale (who did the rating was not reported). The five-point scales were pathological at both extremes, and the authors' interpretation that the results implied hyperactivity and short attention are thus problematical.

   The sibling comparisons (Table 12.8) generated similar results. However, in this sib-pair analysis, it is possible that mothers may have avoided smoking in a subsequent pregnancy *because* their former child had manifested problems. In addition, other kinds of stress may vary between pregnancies and

**Table 12.7** Standardized regression coefficient at age seven with number of cigarettes/day during pregnancy, adjusted for several factors

|  | Regression coefficient |
|---|---|
| Spelling[1] | −0.046*** |
| Reading[1] | −0.042* |
| Arithmetic[1] | −0.020 |
| Attention span[2] | −0.049*** |
| Activity level[2] | 0.043* |

* $P < 0.05$; *** $P < 0.001$.
[1] Wide range achievement test scores.
[2] Five-point scale.

From Naeye and Peters (1984). NCPP population at Boston Lying-In Hospital (482); subset of 2903 white infants in middle of SES rank, and 578 same-sex sibling pairs (presumably from all NCPP sites) among whom mother smoked only in one pregnancy, balanced for birth order.

**Table 12.8** Achievement scores among 7-year-old children of 2903 white middle socio-economic status women, unadjusted results

|  | Smoking during pregnancy (cigarettes/day) | | |
|---|---|---|---|
|  | 0 | 1–19 | 20+ |
| Spelling[1] | 27.4 | 27.0 | 26.6*** |
| Reading[1] | 41.0 | 39.8 | 39.2*** |
| Arithmetic[1] | 21.6 | 21.5 | 21.1*** |

*** $P < 0.001$.
[1] Wide range achievement test scores.

From Naeye and Peters (1984). NCPP population at Boston Lying-In Hospital (482); subset of 2903 white infants in middle of SES rank, and 578 same-sex sibling pairs (presumably from all NCPP sites) among whom mother smoked only in one pregnancy, balanced for birth order.

**Table 12.9** Sibling comparisons, test scores at age
seven (578 pairs)

| | Mother smoked during pregnancy | |
|---|---|---|
| | No | Yes |
| Spelling[1] | 24.80 | 24.00* |
| Reading[1] | 36.00 | 34.20** |
| Arithmetic[1] | 20.50 | 20.10 |
| Attention span[2] | 2.95 | 2.90* |
| Motor activity[2] | 2.91 | 2.98* |

* $P < 0.05$; ** $P < 0.01$.
[1] Wide range achievement test scores.
[2] Five-point scale.
　From Naeye and Peters (1984). NCPP populations at Boston
Lying-In Hospital (482); subset of 2903 white infants in middle of
SES rank, and 578 same-sex sibling pairs (presumably from all NCPP
sites) among whom mother smoked only in one pregnancy, balanced
for birth order.

might have led both to the mother's smoking in either pregnancy and to
circumstances that were detrimental to the child's development. In spite of
these limitations, the results for cognition were impressive, as static environmental, maternal, and familial circumstances (mother's height, intelligence,
etc.) would be similar for both sibs. The results for abnormal behaviour
(activity and attention) were less convincing; the five-point scales were patho-
logic at both extremes and mean differences on the scales cannot directly be
interpreted as demonstrating pathology.

## Seattle longitudinal study

Martin *et al.* (1977) reported the first of a series of papers following a cohort of
children born to predominantly white middle-class pregnant women recruited
at two Seattle hospitals. The sample was weighted to over-represent mothers
who were heavy smokers and users of alcohol. Two learning tasks were presented to 2-day-old infants. Sixty-three were tested on a head turning task and
80 on two sucking learning tasks. There was a significant relationship between
maternal cigarette smoking and less efficient performance on the head turning
task, with a significant interaction between alcohol and tobacco use. The
magnitude of differences was not reported. On the sucking task, babies born
to mothers who smoked and did not drink did better than controls, while
combined maternal alcohol and nicotine consumption was associated with
poor neonatal performance. The results were presented qualitatively.
　Streissguth *et al.* (1980) studied 462 8-month-old infants in the Seattle

study. There was no suggestion of relationship between maternal smoking on either the Bayley mental development index or the Bayley psychomotor development index. The same group presented a laboratory vigilance task to 475 of these children between ages of 6 and 8 months (Streissguth *et al.* 1986). There was no relationship with cigarette use.

Landesman-Dwyer *et al.* (1981) studied 128 4-year-olds from the same longitudinal study in Seattle. Maternal cigarette smoking during pregnancy was unrelated to any subscale of the Caldwell HOME scale, or to any of eight specific behaviour patterns assessed at meal- and story-time. Mothers ranked their children on 98 items, describing the child's temperament. The offspring of smokers showed significant differences in three groups of items:

(1) greater willingness to approach strangers in novel situations;
(2) greater persistence, interpreted both as stubbornness and sustained involvement in single activities;
(3) greater intensity, interpreted as a more negative reaction when upset, annoyed or disciplined.

In this study, children of smokers were thus not regarded as being inattentive.

In 1984 Streissguth *et al.* reported on a vigilance task amongst the same cohort (452 singletons) but at the age of four. Children of smokers during pregnancy made significantly more errors of omission, had a significantly lower ratio of correct to total responses, and had fewer trials in which they were oriented. There was no significant relationship between maternal smoking and reaction time nor to time moving during the testing session. The results were adjusted for birth order, maternal alcohol and caffeine use, education, and nutrition. Adjustment for age and sex did not affect results. The magnitude of the deficits associated with tobacco use, and the impact of adjustment procedures, are unclear from the presentation. While it was stated that Caldwell's HOME score at age one was not associated with alcohol and nicotine use, it is not clear whether any attempts have been made to include assessment of the current home environment in the analysis of development at age four.

## Ottowa Prenatal Prospective Study

Gusella and Fried (1983), in the first of a series of reports from the Ottawa Prenatal Prospective Study, assessed 84 13-month-olds. Detailed data had been gathered three times during pregnancy, on cigarettes smoked, other substances used, and a variety of background factors. The only significant relationship of maternal smoking during pregnancy with any aspect of the Bayley tests, after adjustment for father's education, was with a set of items that the investigators grouped under the rubric of verbal comprehension. Two other sets of indices were related to cigarette consumption *prior* to pregnancy, the psychomotor development index, and an item cluster called fine motor skills (Table 12.10).

Three further reports were published about this cohort in 1987 (Fried and Makin 1987; Fried *et al.* 1987; Fried and O'Connell 1987). It was initially reported that there was no relationship between cigarette smoking during pregnancy and somatic growth at 12 or 24 months. Later, Fried and Watkinson (1988) reported quantitative results and found a 1.6 cm decrement in height at 12 months of age and a 1.1 cm decrement in head circumference at 24 months of age, both significant. They did not report differences in height at 24 months nor head circumference at 12 months; presumably neither of these was significantly different. They only reported the contrast between heavy smokers (15 mg nicotine/day) and non-smokers, and no results were presented for children of intermediate level smokers. In the neonatal period maternal smoking was associated with reduced infant habituation to sound (a direction opposite to that reported in other studies) and increased tremulousness.

The Bayley mental development index at 12 months of age was significantly lower amongst the children of smokers, 96.5 versus 109.5. The unadjusted means were equally divergent at 24 months, but these were no longer significantly different. (The numbers of children of smokers in each of these analyses was only 23 and 22, respectively.) The meaning of these large

**Table 12.10** Maternal nicotine consumption before and during pregnancy correlated with Bayley examinations at 13 months

|  | Development index | | Item clusters[1] | | |
|---|---|---|---|---|---|
|  | Mental | Psychomotor | Verbal comprehension | Spoken language | Fine motor |
| Pre-pregnancy consumption | −0.20* | −0.37*** | −0.27** | −0.05 | −0.27** |
| +adjustment for father's education | −0.13 | −0.35** | −0.16 | — | −0.21* |
| Pregnancy consumption | −0.06 | −0.19* | −0.31** | −0.05 | −0.18 |
| +adjustment for father's education | −0.03 | −0.15 | −0.22* | — | −0.11 |

— not presented.
* $P < 0.05$; ** $P < 0.01$; *** $P < 0.001$.
[1] A priori regrouping of items from Bayley exam.
  From Gusella and Fried (1983). Prospective Study—13-month-olds who were products of 84 consecutive pregnancies, 11/78 to 12/79. Data on cigarette use (and other factors) gathered at three times during pregnancy.

differences was called into some question by the fact that the Caldwell HOME inventory, an index of the learning environment to which the child was exposed, was highly significantly negatively related to mother's smoking.

A vigilance task modified from Streissguth *et al.* (1986) was applied to these children when they were 4 to 7 years of age (Kristjansson *et al.* 1989). The authors chose to use different statistical tests for different outcomes, and reported only significant differences. They found that maternal nicotine use was associated with a significantly increased increment in variance in child activity, but not for omission errors. When studying commission errors on the vigilance test, they used a different criterion, the increase in goodness of fit chi-square. The increase of goodness of fit for auditory but not visual commission errors was significant. Why the results for commission errors and omission errors were presented with different statistical models was not explained. Mother's education was reported to be strongly correlated to cigarette smoking during pregnancy ($r = -0.336$; $P < 0.001$) but mother's education was not adjusted in the early results of this series of studies. Further, birth weight and maternal weight gain were sometimes used as control variables: maternal weight gain in analyses of somatic growth and neurological status, and birth weight in the analysis of neurological status. As both birth weight (almost surely) and maternal weight gain (in all likelihood) are depressed by cigarette smoking, the results were probably overcontrolled and possible effects of smoking would have been understated.

## Other studies in chronological order of publication

Wingerd and Schoen (1974) demonstrated highly significant depression of height among 5-year-olds from the Kaiser Permanente Clinic in Oakland, California, whose mothers smoked during pregnancy. Results were controlled for sex; birth order; length of gestation; parental age, education, income, and stature; mother's age at menarche; and father's occupational status. The height at age five of the children whose mothers smoked less than 15 cigarettes per day was depressed 0.40 cm, compared with children of non-smokers, and of those who smoked more than that, 0.90 cm.

Denson *et al.* (1975) matched 20 hyperkinetic (methylphenidate-sensitive) 5- to 15-year-old children for social class, age, and sex with one dyslexic and one normal control. The average number of cigarettes smoked in pregnancy was significantly higher among mothers of subjects, 14.3 per cent compared with 6.0 and 6.3 per cent in the respective control groups. The difference was even more marked when considering the number currently smoked, 23.3 per cent in the hyperkinetic group compared with 6.1 and 8.1 per cent in the two control groups. There was no significant association with paternal smoking.

Dunn *et al.* (1976, 1977) studied all traceable 6½-year-old survivors born at the Vancouver General Hospital between September 1958 and March 1965 with birth weights under 4½ pounds (plus several referred low birth weight children). Controls were normal birth weight subjects recruited at the end of the study period, chosen from non-paying patients in an attempt to control for social disparity, as low birth weight occurs more often among those of lower status. Results were presented within birth weight and gestational strata. From the reported results, it is not possible to judge how successful was this control strategy.

We used their combined published data to calculate differences in outcome between children of smokers and non-smokers, making the assumption that 4 per cent of births weighed under 4½ pounds. Children of smokers were significantly shorter (2.02 cm; $P < 0.001$) and had significantly lower full-scale Wechsler Intelligence Scale for Children (WISC) performance IQ (Table 12.11).

However, Bender Gestalt, Knox cubes, sentence repetition, and draw-a-person were not significantly different. Although the overall verbal IQ was not significantly different, children of smokers did significantly worse on three subscales—block completion, coding, and vocabulary. In the same study teachers had reported misbehaviour to be more common among boys whose mothers had smoked during pregnancy (but not significantly according to the tabulated data) on the Haggerty–Olson–Wickman Behaviour Rating Schedule. There were significant relationships of maternal smoking to lower cognition,

**Table 12.11** Estimated length/height (cm) in babies born in the Vancouver General Hospital by maternal smoking habit in pregnancy

|  | Length/height (cm)[1] | | |
|  | Non-smokers | Smokers | Difference |
| --- | --- | --- | --- |
| Age |  |  |  |
| Birth | 50.90 | 50.39 | 0.51 |
| 1 year | 75.36 | 74.44 | 0.92* |
| 4 years | 103.19 | 101.51 | 1.68** |
| 6.5 years | 119.09 | 117.07 | 2.02*** |
| Psychological status, age 6.5[1] |  |  |  |
| WISC IQ |  |  |  |
| Verbal performance | 109.7 | 104.6 | 5.1* |
| full scale | 109.9 | 105.9 | 4.0* |
| vocal encoding | −0.50 | −0.73 | −0.23* |

[1] Calculated from authors data, assuming rate of birth $< 2041$ g bw $= 4\%$.
* $P < 0.05$; ** $P < 0.01$; *** $P < 0.001$.

From Dunn *et al.* (1976, 1977). All infants born at Vancouver General Hospital $< 2041$ g birth weight from 9/58 to 3/65 ($n = 480$) + 17 born elsewhere. 205 controls $> 2500$ g birth weight; 'non-pay' patients, recruited in 1965–66; 234 low birth weight, 146 full birth weight followed to 6.5 years.

poorer physical traits, retarded social development, and less stable temperament.

Saxon (1978) found four of twenty items on the Brazelton Assessment Scale to be significantly different in 15 4- to 6-day-old infants whose mothers had smoked 15 or more cigarettes per day, compared to 17 controls 'matched' for maternal age, social class, and parity. There was no explanation how there could be more 'matched' controls than cases, nor was it stated whether the observer was blind to the child's study status. The author interpreted the direction of all four differences to be adverse, but the tabulated data indicated that infants of smokers habituated more rapidly to an auditory stimulus, a response usually assumed to be positively correlated with later intelligence.

Hingson *et al.* (1982) related 1 and 5 min Apgar scores to amount of cigarette smoking during pregnancy, assessed by postpartum interview. They found no significant relationships between Apgar scores and cigarette smoking. No numerical results were presented.

Picone *et al.* (1982) studied 60 pregnant women and their offspring. The population was probably stratified by weight gain during pregnancy, but this was not specified in the publication. They found that Apgar scores were not significantly related to smoking, but that maternal smoking was related to more rapid auditory habituation and less good auditory orientation, autonomic regulation, and regulation of state, by Brazelton examinations performed at 2 and 3 days of age. While performance scores were abnormal at 2 and 3 days of age, they were not at 2 weeks. The description of the analytic methods left unclear whether maternal weight and smoking might have been confounded either by the sampling design or in analysis. What and how possible confounding was addressed was not specified.

Rantakallio (1983) compared 1763 14-year-old children whose mothers had smoked during pregnancy to 1781 children whose mothers had not smoked, matched by maternal marital status, age, parity, and place of residence. The children whose mothers smoked under 10 cigarettes a day during pregnancy were 0.6 cm shorter than children of non-smokers, and those of women who smoked 10 or more cigarettes a day were 0.9 cm shorter. These results were reported to be significant with value of $P = 0.013$, by analysis of covariance adjusting for maternal height and age, number of older and younger sibs, father's social class, and sex of child. After further adjustment for several adverse maternal factors, as well as paternal smoking, the difference was no longer significant, but control for paternal smoking may have caused the relationship with maternal smoking to be underestimated. Ability on theoretical school subjects was significantly depressed among children of smokers, and remained significantly depressed even after further adjustment for the adverse maternal factors and paternal smoking.

Jacobson *et al.* (1984) performed the Brazelton examination on days 3 and/or 4 of life on 173 infants of predominantly white, middle-class mothers. In this study maternal smoking was associated with lower irritability

$(0.05 < P < 0.10)$ and less good auditory orientation $(0.05 < P < 0.10)$. This latter result was entirely accounted for by adjusting for socio-economic status and caffeine use. This project was impressive for the careful attention that was paid to potential confounding between smoking, alcohol, and caffeine use of the mother.

Fox *et al.* (1990) and Sexton *et al.* (1990) studied 754 singleton children whose mothers had been participants in a randomized trial of smoking cessation during pregnancy. They found a decrement in height of 1.13 cm among children whose mothers smoked during pregnancy, which changed only marginally after adjusting for social class and postpartum smoking, but was more than halved with adjustment for birth weight and duration of gestation. One-third of the significant unadjusted increment in weight was lost after socioeconomic status and postpartum smoking adjustment: no difference remained after accounting for perinatal status. They found a decrement of 0.41 in the McCarthy general cognitive index associated with maternal smoking during pregnancy, which remained highly significant at 0.37 after adjustment for potential confounding factors, and 0.34 after adjusting additionally for fetal growth. The memory and motor scales of the McCarthy were no longer significantly different after adjusting for confounding factors. The original experimental design was not used in this analysis, and the power of randomization to equalize social differences across groups was not utilized. The relatively small changes in smoking effects with adjustment for confounding factors suggests that the array of information used may have been less than fully descriptive of the differences in the child's learning environment that have usually been associated with maternal smoking.

In Newcastle, Kolvin *et al.* (personal communication) studied 59 5- to 7-year-old children of short gestation (the criterion was not stated) 139 of whom were light-for dates, and 186 children of normal gestation and birth weight. In three of four subgroups, children of smokers (5+ cigarettes/day) had a lower language quotient, and in one of four, IQ or Rutter behaviour scores, more than two units worse than control children. No statistical tests of these differences were reported. After controlling for social class and maternal neuroticism, children of smokers did significantly worse on 11 of 72 items measuring behaviour and temperament, six of 25 indices of cognitive function, and 13 of 24 'physical' measures (height, weight, and unspecified neurological indices). With further control for birth weight, there was no change in the number of significant behavioural and temperamental differences, but only two cognitive measures and no physical measures remained significant. Thus, prenatal growth retardation entirely mediated the associations of maternal smoking with physical measures, partly mediated those with cognitive function, but played no part in the association with behavioural functions. Of the behavioural dimensions 'acting out' and hyperactivity were significantly related to maternal smoking (both $P < 0.001$), and effects were undiminished by statistical control for social class or maternal neuroticism.

The effects were entirely contributed by the children of short gestation or whose birthweight was below the < 5th percentile for their gestational age. Also, among the very small for dates, smoking was significantly related to misconduct, and negatively to shyness, and these differences were again unaffected by the same control variables.

## Physical stature and postnatal parental smoking

Rona *et al.* (1981) related height among primary school children to the number of adult smokers in the child's household, separately for England and Scotland, from the National Study of Health and Growth. Smoking in pregnancy was accounted for in analysis by adjusting for reported birth weight. There were significant relationships between the number of adult smokers in the household and childhood stature in England, which were reduced, but not eliminated, by adjustment for birth weight and social class; differences in the smaller Scottish sample were not significant after such adjustment.

## Discussion

### Somatic development and maternal smoking during pregnancy

There is a consistent decrement of around 1–2 cm in children's height associated with maternal smoking during pregnancy. The first report from the Ottawa study (Fried and O'Connell 1987) found no significant relationship, but in a more recent communication there were several significant relationships (Fried and Watkinson 1988). In the National Child Development Study adjustment for social status and several other variables accounted for about 40 per cent of the difference in height between children of smokers and non-smokers, before controlling for birth weight. The exact extent to which the remaining deficit was due to smoking remains uncertain, but the consistency and persistence of these findings after statistical adjustment for possible confounding variables suggests a causal relationship. However, whether such depressed stature has functional consequences remains an open question.

### Mental development, neurological status and behaviour, and maternal smoking

*Neonatal effects*   The case for a relationship between maternal smoking during pregnancy and neonatal neurological status and behaviour is mixed, and is reviewed here because of possible implications for later cognition and behaviour. The only studies in which Apgar scores appeared related to maternal smoking during pregnancy were those of Garn *et al.* (1980, 1981). Among whites, the effect was limited to the few infants whose mothers smoked over two packs of cigarettes a day and, among blacks, over one pack a day. It is therefore not surprising that other investigators have not observed a positive relationship between maternal smoking during pregnancy and Apgar score: very few studies had enough very heavy smokers to retest this observation.

Reported relationships between maternal smoking during pregnancy and abnormalities in the Brazelton neonatal behavioural assessment scale have been mixed. Generally, neonates of smoking mothers oriented less well to auditory stimuli. Saxon (1978) found infants of smoking mothers less easily consolable, but did not note any state difference associated with maternal smoking, while Picone *et al.* (1982) observed poor autonomic regulation and regulation of state among infants of smokers. On the other hand, they found that performance scores, which were depressed at 2 and 3 days of age, were normal by 2 weeks. Possibly the early abnormalities on the Brazelton exam were associated with effects of withdrawal from toxic cigarette products and may or may not have long-term implications. Jacobson *et al.* (1984) noted *lower* irritability among infants of smoking mothers (at the margins of statistical significance) as well as less good auditory orientation, consistent with most other studies. Fried and Makin (1987) found significantly reduced habituation to sound among infants of smokers (as well as increased tremulousness). Results on auditory habituation were mixed, as both Saxon (1978) and Picone *et al.* (1982) found increased auditory habituation, in contrast to the results of Fried and Makin (1987).

Thus, there do not appear to be dramatic, or even consistent behavioural effects on the neonate from the smoking of their mothers other than less good auditory orientation. Whether such possible effects are associated with any long-term or permanent deficit is unknown.

*Infant cognitive and motor development*   The evidence for deficits in infant development revealed by the use of the Bayley tests associated with maternal smoking is inconsistent. Garn *et al.* (1980, 1981) showed weak trends of increased rates of low Bayley scores among whites with increased amounts of smoking, with the highest rates of abnormality among white infants in the few whose mothers had smoked more than two packs of cigarettes a day. There was little or no relationship of smoking among black mothers with the Bayley motor scores of their infants, and a weak relationship with the Bayley mental score. Streissguth *et al.* (1980) could not demonstrate a relationship between prenatal maternal smoking and either the Bayley mental or psychomotor developmental indices in the Seattle longitudinal study. Gusella and Fried (1983) found non-significant relationships between cigarette smoking during pregnancy and either the Bayley mental or psychomotor index at 13 months of age, but a strong and highly significant relationship between the psychomotor developmental index and amount of cigarette smoking *prior* to pregnancy. Later, studying the same children, Fried and Watkinson (1988) reported a significant decrement in the Bayley mental developmental index at 12 months of age associated with smoking during pregnancy. The strongest set of relationships in the preschool period were those reported by Sexton *et al.* (1990), with a mean decrement in the McCarthy general cognitive index at 3 years of age of about one-third of a standard unit ($P < 0.01$). On the other hand, adjustment for their set of potential confounding covariates accounted for less variance than in any of the other reported studies, and it is therefore an open question how well they described the array of social characteristics that have typically been observed in the families of American children whose mothers smoke. Thus, there was no consistent nor strong pattern of deficit in infant or preschool child development among offspring of smoking mothers.

*Cognitive development and achievement in school age children, and maternal smoking in pregnancy* There is a consistent pattern of depressed cognitive development and school achievement associated with maternal smoking during pregnancy. In very small studies in which differences might not have reached statistical significance, there were regular and consistent patterns of lower IQ and ability, and less advanced verbal, reading, and mathematical skills associated with maternal smoking during pregnancy. On the other hand, it appears beyond current knowledge to conclude that these associations were causally related to maternal smoking.

Much the same problem arises in attempting to relate starvation in early life to later behaviour and function (Rush 1984). One insult cannot be presumed to exist independent of a web of other contingent and powerful influences on the child. When social class has been taken into account, differences in cognition and achievement between children of smokers and of non-smokers are markedly attenuated; for instance, differences were about halved among 11-year-olds in the National Child Development Study with social class adjustment (Butler and Goldstein 1973). Thus, any secure judgement on these issues must be withheld, and further research awaited. The sibling comparisons of Naeye and Peters (1984) represents the strongest attempt to overcome these inherent methodologic problems.

*Behaviour, temperament, and hyperactivity* There appear to be consistent character, temperamental, and behavioural difficulties among children whose mothers smoked during pregnancy. Denson *et al.* (1975) found that mothers of hyperactive children smoked much more than controls both during pregnancy, and later. Dunn *et al.* (1976) found that children of smokers, especially males, were judged worse by teachers on all components of the Haggerty–Olson–Wickman Behaviour Rating. These children had more frequent misbehaviour (although this was not statistically significant), depressed cognition, worse social development, more frequent problems of temperament, and more abnormal physical traits. Streissguth *et al.* (1984) found amount of maternal cigarette smoking in pregnancy significantly related to poor performance by 4-year-olds on a vigilance task. There was no observed effect of maternal cigarette smoking on a vigilance task among the same children at ages 6½ to 8½ (personal communication). It is not clear that the ratings reported by Naeye and Peters (1984) represented abnormal levels of activity or inattention, since the scales used were pathological at both extremes. Kolvin *et al.* (personal communication) found 11 of 72 behavioural and temperamental indices significantly different (presumably worse in children of mothers who smoked) and these differences appeared to be unaffected by adjusting for the disparity in birth weight between children of smokers and non-smokers. Davie *et al.* (1972) found social adjustment in the former significantly worse at age seven. Nichols and Chen (1981) demonstrated a marked association of maternal smoking with all three components of what they termed minimal brain damage at age seven: learning difficulties, hyperactivity–impulsivity, and neurological soft signs.

In sum, the reported differences are consistent, particularly for hyperactivity. However, the evidence that maternal smoking during pregnancy is causally related to abnormal behaviour is not entirely convincing. Are the abnormalities caused by smoking, or do they reflect other differences in the lives of children of smokers? In the sibling comparisons, did smoking reflect stresses present around the time of one pregnancy, but not the other? Whether maternal smoking during pregnancy causes later behavioural abnormality in the child remains an important and intriguing hypothesis, but from the available data it is not possible to judge whether a causal relationship exists.

## Acknowledgement

This work was supported by NICHD Grant R01-HD13347.

## References

Broman, S. H., Nichols, P. L., and Kennedy, W. A. (1975). *Preschool IQ: prenatal and early developmental correlates*. Lawrence Erlbaum Associates, Hillsdale, New Jersey.

Butler, N. R. and Alberman, E. D. (1969). *Perinatal problems: the second report of the 1958 British Perinatal Mortality Survey*. Livingstone, Edinburgh.

Butler, N. R. and Bonham, D. G. (1963). *Perinatal mortality: the first report of the 1958 British Perinatal Mortality Survey*. Livingstone, Edinburgh.

Butler, N. R. and Goldstein, H. (1973). Smoking in pregnancy and subsequent child development. *British Medical Journal*, **4**, 573–5.

Davie, R., Butler, N. R., and Goldstein, H. (1972). *From birth to seven: a report of the National Child Development Study*. Longman, London.

Denson, R., Nanso, J. L., and McWatters, R. N. (1975). Hyperkinesis and maternal smoking. *Canadian Psychiatric Association Journal*, **20**, 183–7.

Dunn, H. G., McBurney, A. K., Ingram, S., and Hunter, C. M. (1976). Maternal cigarette smoking during pregnancy and the child's subsequent development: I.

Physical growth to the age of 6½ years. *Canadian Journal of Public Health*, **67**, 499–505.

Dunn, H. G., McBurney, S. K., Ingram, S., and Hunter, C. M. (1977). Maternal cigarette smoking during pregnancy and the child's subsequent development: II. Neurological and intellectual maturation to the age of 6½ years. *Canadian Journal of Public Health*, **68**, 43–50.

Fogelman, K. (1980). Smoking in pregnancy and subsequent development of the child. *Child: Care, Health and Development*, **6**, 233–49.

Fox, N. L., Sexton, M., and Hebel, J. R. (1990). Prenatal exposure to tobacco: I. Effects on physical growth at age three. *International Journal of Epidemiology*, **19**, 66–71.

Fried, P. A. and Makin, J. E. (1987). Neonatal behavioral correlates of prenatal exposure to marihuana, cigarettes and alcohol in a low risk population. *Neurotoxicology and Teratology*, **9**, 1–7.

Fried, P. A. and O'Connell, C. M. (1987). A comparison of the effects of prenatal exposure to tobacco, alcohol, cannabis and caffeine on birth size and subsequent growth. *Neurotoxicology and Teratology*, **9**, 79–85.

Fried, P. A. and Watkinson, B. (1988). 12- and 24-month neurobehavioural follow-up of children prenatally exposed to marihuana, cigarettes and alcohol. *Neurotoxicology and Teratology*, **10**, 305–13.

Fried, P. A., Watkinson, B., Dillon, R. F., and Dulberg, C. S. (1987). Neonatal neurological status in a low-risk population after prenatal exposure to cigarettes, marijuana, and alcohol. *Developmental and Behavioral Pediatrics*, **8**, 318–26.

Garn, S. M., Petzold, A. S., Ridella, S. A., and Johnston, M. (1980). Effect of smoking during pregnancy on Apgar and Bayley scores. *Lancet*, **ii**, 912–13.

Garn, S. M., Johnston, M., Ridella, S. A., and Retzold, A. S. (1981). Effect of maternal cigarette smoking on Apgar scores. *American Journal of Diseases in Children*, **135**, 503–6.

Gusella, J. L. and Fried, P. A. (1983). Effects of maternal social drinking and smoking on offspring at 13 months. *Neurobehavioral Toxicology and Teratology*, **6**, 13–17.

Hardy, J. B. and Mellits, E. D. (1972). Does maternal smoking during pregnancy have a long-term effect on the child? *Lancet*, **ii**, 1332–6.

Harrison, R. H. and Kass, E. H. (1967). Differences between Negro and white pregnant women on the MMPI. *Journal of Consulting Clinical Psychology*, **31**, 454–63.

Heath, C. W. (1958). Differences between smokers and nonsmokers. *Archives of Internal Medicine*, **101**, 377–88.

Hingson, R., Gould, J. B., Morelock, S., Kayne, H., Heeren, T., Alpert, J. J., *et al.* (1982). Maternal cigarette smoking, psychoactive substance use, and infant Apgar scores. *American Journal of Obstetrics and Gynecology*, **144**, 959–66.

Jacobson, W. W., Fein, G. G., Jacobson, J. L., Schwartz, P. M., and Dowler, J. K. (1984). Neonatal correlates of prenatal exposure to smoking, caffeine, and alcohol. *Infant Behavior and Development*, **7**, 253–65.

Kristjansson, E. A., Fried, P. A., and Watkinson, B. (1989). Maternal smoking during pregnancy affects children's vigilance performance. *Drug and Alcohol Dependence*, **24**, 11–19.

Landesman-Dwyer, S., Ragozin, A. S., and Little, R. E. (1981). Behavioral correlates of prenatal alcohol exposure: A four year follow-up study. *Neurobehavioral Toxicology and Teratology*, **3**, 187–93.

Lilienfeld, A. M. (1959). Emotional and other selected characteristics of cigarette smokers and nonsmokers as related to epidemiological studies of lung cancer and other diseases. *Journal of the National Cancer Institute*, **22**, 259–82.

Martin, J., Martin, D. C., Lund, C. A., and Streissguth, A. P. (1977). Maternal alcohol ingestion and cigarette smoking and their effects on newborn conditioning. *Alcoholism: Clinical and Experimental Research*, **1**, 243–7.

Naeye, R. L. (1981). Influence of maternal cigarette smoking during pregnancy on fetal and childhood growth. *Obstetrics and Gynecology*, **57**, 18–21.

Naeye, R. L. and Peters, E. C. (1984). Mental development of children whose mothers smoked during pregnancy. *Journal of the American College of Obstetrics and Gynecology*, **64**, 601–7.

Nichols, P. L. and Chen, T. C. (1981). *Minimal brain dysfunction: a prospective study*. Lawrence Erlbaum Associates, Hillsdale, New Jersey.

Picone, T. A., Allen, L. H., Olsen, P. N., and Ferris, M. E. (1982). Pregnancy outcome in North American women. II. Effects of diet, cigarette smoking, stress, and weight gain on placentas, and on neonatal physical and behavioral characteristics. *American Journal of Clinical Nutrition*, **36**, 1214–24.

Rantakallio, P. (1983). A follow-up study up to the age of 14 of children whose mothers smoked during pregnancy. *Acta Paediatrica Scandinavica*, **72**, 747–53.

Reiter, H. H. (1970). Some EPPS differences between smokers and nonsmokers. *Perception and Motor Skills*, **30**, 253.

Rona, R. J., Florey, C. D., Clarke, G. C., and Chinn, S. (1981). Parental smoking at home and height of children. *British Medical Journal*, **23**, 1363.

Rush, D. (1984). The behavioral consequences of protein-energy deprivation and supplementation in early life: An epidemiologic perspective. In *Nutrition and behavior, vol. 5, human nutrition: a comprehensive treatise*, (ed. J. R. Galler), pp. 119–58. Plenum Press, New York.

Rush, D. and Callahan, K. R. (1989). Exposure to passive cigarette smoking and child development: A critical review. *Annals of the New York Academy of Sciences*, **562**, 74–100.

Rush, D. and Kass, E. H. (1972). Maternal smoking: A reassessment of the association with perinatal mortality. *American Journal of Epidemiology*, **96**, 183–96.

Saxon, D. W. (1978). The behaviour of infants whose mothers smoke in pregnancy. *Early Human Development*, **2**, 363–9.

Schneider, N. G. and Houston, J. P. (1970). Smoking and anxiety. *Psychological Reports*, **26**, 941.

Sexton, M., Fox, N. L., and Hebel, J. R. (1990). Prenatal exposure to tobacco: II Effects on cognitive functioning at age three. *International Journal of Epidemiology*, **19**, 72–7.

Streissguth, A. O., Barr, H. M., Martin, D. C., and Herman, C. S. (1980). Effects of maternal alcohol, nicotine, and caffeine use during pregnancy on infant mental and motor development at eight months. *Alcoholism: Clinical and Experimental Research*, **4**, 152–74.

Streissguth, A. P., Martin, D. C., Barr, H. M., and Sandman, B. M. (1984). Intrauterine alcohol and nicotine exposure: Attention and reaction time in 4-year-old children. *Developmental Psychology*, **20**, 533–41.

Streissguth, A. P., Barr, H. M., Sampson, P. D., Parrish-Johnson, J. C., Kirchner, G. L., and Martrin, D. C. (1986). Attention, distraction and reaction time at age 7 years and prenatal alcohol exposure. *Neurobehavioral Toxicology and Teratology*, **8**, 717–25.

Wingerd, J. and Schoen, E. J. (1974). Factors influencing length at birth and height at five years. *Pediatrics*, **53**, 737–41.

# 13. Prevention of smoking in pregnancy: results of intervention

*Christine MacArthur and George Knox*

## Introduction

Smoking during pregnancy has been shown repeatedly to be associated with adverse outcomes of pregnancy, in particular with reduced birth weight and corresponding higher rates of perinatal mortality (Butler *et al.* 1972; Surgeon General 1980). The early findings all came from observational studies comparing smokers with non-smokers and ex-smokers. These groups, however, might be different in ways other than their smoking and it was not certain that the associations were causal. Only a randomized intervention, demonstrating that increased birth weight results directly from persuading pregnant smokers to reduce their smoking, would allow a firm inference that the association was causal (Butler *et al.* 1972); and at the same time indicate the pragmatic value of the intervention.

Donovan (1977) was the first to conduct a study with an experimental design to examine the effect of an anti-smoking intervention in pregnancy on subsequent birth weight. The women in his study were randomly allocated to a test group and a control group, the former receiving intensive anti-smoking advice from a doctor at each antenatal visit. Although there was a reported significant reduction in smoking in the test group compared with controls, there was no difference in the mean birth weight of babies in the two groups. Donovan suggested, *inter alia*, that stopping smoking after contact with the hospital antenatal service was already too late to prevent a reduction in birth weight.

In 1984 the results of a second trial were reported from the USA (Sexton and Hebel 1984). This trial showed a positive result: there was a significant reduction of 92 g in mean birth weight and 0.6 cm in mean length of the control group compared with the treatment group.

In Birmingham in 1982 a randomized trial had commenced to answer the same question as these earlier studies: can the size of the infant at birth be increased by persuading a group of pregnant women to reduce their smoking? It had the additional aim of determining whether this could be achieved within the context of routine antenatal care and existing resources (MacArthur *et al.* 1987).

## Subjects and methods

All women who were smokers at the time of their antenatal booking at one Birmingham hospital, within a 12-month period, were included in the trial. These smokers were allocated to the intervention or the control group according to the date of their booking visit, using a 4-weekly block alternation. For logistic reasons individual randomization was not practical.

A total of 1259 smokers were originally enrolled into the trial, with 1156 of these proceeding to delivery in the same hospital. The remainder miscarried, moved out of the area or rebooked in other hospitals.

Those women allocated to the intervention group received specially designed supplementary anti-smoking health education, whilst the women in the control group received only the advice contained within routine antenatal care. Routine care sometimes included advice about smoking, but it was minimal and irregular. It was considered unethical—and in the event proved unnecessary—to remove such routinely offered advice from controls. Data were later obtained from the controls to assess what this had in practice comprised.

The planned supplementary health education was to be given by the obstetrician to the women in the intervention group in the course of the booking examination. The women were to be advised by the obstetrician that they should stop smoking for the remainder of their pregnancy and told about the effects of cigarette smoking on the fetus. An opportunity was to be given for questions or discussion and a specially designed leaflet was handed to the women to support the verbal advice. As a back-up, if the obstetricians omitted to give the full planned intervention, the midwives were requested to do so instead. The women were not told that a trial was in progress or that they were included in it: or that the advice given was other than routine.

At the time of the intervention, the only information obtained from the women was about their smoking habits since becoming pregnant. The main data collection occurred later, after delivery and before discharge from the hospital, when a member of the research team interviewed both the intervention and the control groups, using an identical data schedule. The women were told that the study was about various forms of health-related advice commonly given to women during pregnancy, and the effects of such advice upon their behaviour. Particular interest was to be focused on advice about smoking. A detailed description of smoking throughout pregnancy was obtained, and of advice and information received by the women from all sources, including the hospital antenatal staff. Data on infant size and other relevant clinical details, as well as maternal age, height, parity, and paternal social class, were extracted from the maternal case-notes.

Of the 1156 smokers recruited and delivered in the hospital, 1008 (87 per cent) were finally interviewed. The others were missed mainly because of isolations for infection, early discharges, and difficulties in tracing due to change of name subsequent to recruitment. None refused to be interviewed. Twin deliveries (six cases, eight controls) were then removed from the study and a further twelve women (eight cases, four controls) had to be excluded because it was not possible to trace their case-notes. The final analysis was based on 982 smokers at booking, 493 in the intervention group and 489 in the control group.

# Results

## Comparison of groups

Table 13.1 shows that the characteristics of the women in the intervention and control groups, as obtained from case notes were generally similar. The only exception was for maternal height; the intervention group contained a smaller proportion of tall women. Additional compared factors included frequency of

**Table 13.1** Characteristics of intervention and control groups

| Variables | Intervention ($n = 493$) | Controls ($n = 489$) |
|---|---|---|
| Mean age at booking (years) | 25.1 (5.1) | 25.4 (5.4) |
| Social class* (%) | | |
|    I, II | 10 | 10 |
|    III | 57 | 57 |
|    IV, V | 25 | 24 |
|    Unclassified | 8 | 9 |
| Education obtained, GCE 'O' and above (%) | 24 | 23 |
| Parity | | |
|    0 | 38 | 40 |
|    1+ | 33 | 31 |
| Mean gestation at booking (weeks) | 15.1 (5.8) | 15.5 (5.3) |
| Mean height (cm)† | 160.4 (6.3) | 161.5 (6.3) |
| Mean number of cigarettes smoked | | |
|    Before pregnancy | 18.6 (8.4) | 17.8 (8.8) |
|    At booking | 14.4 (9.0) | 13.7 (8.7) |
| Experienced sickness/nausea (%) | 42 | 41 |

Standard deviation, where appropriate, in parentheses.
* This is based on women's own present or previous occupation since data on husband's occupation were only recorded in case-notes for 60% of the sample.
† Significant difference between the two groups $P < 0.01$.

smoking advice from non-hospital sources (e.g. media, husband, friends, GP), smoking among the women's social groups, and previous smoking history. None of these differed between the two groups.

## Implementation of the intervention

A basic design requirement of the proposed intervention, namely that it could be incorporated into routine antenatal care, necessitated the participation of a large number of hospital personnel. A total of 34 obstetricians and six GP Unit doctors were involved, as well as numerous midwives, and much time was spent by the researcher on personal explanation of the study. However, within the setting of a very busy clinic, on the evidence of reports from the women, the intervention was not always conducted as planned. The women were asked in detail about all the advice they had received at the hospital; some recalled advice to stop smoking but without information or discussion on the adverse effects; others recalled advice only to cut down. Some recalled being given the leaflet, others did not. Some had obtained advice from the obstetricians, others from the midwives. The full intervention in its exact planned format (i.e. all components from the obstetrician) was reported by only 10 per cent of the women in the intervention group; but a further 13 per cent had received the full intervention either from the midwife, or from both sources. Full or partial conformity with the intervention plan was recorded for 90 per cent of the group, i.e. 90 per cent recalled receiving some form of advice and/or leaflet, compared with only 58 per cent of the women in the control group (where only 'routine care' was being given).

The completeness of the recalled intervention varied among different categories of women: especially according to parity. Women having first births were much more likely to have received 'adequate' advice (e.g. 61 per cent of primiparae recalled advice to stop smoking completely compared with 45 per cent of multiparae). In the control group there were no parity differences in the content of advice received.

## Smoking behaviour

Although the main outcome measure of this experiment was the size of the infant, a necessary intermediate outcome was the behavioural response to the intervention. In the event of there being no differences in birth weight, assessment would have been made as to whether this was because the planned intervention, although adequately executed, had nevertheless been ineffective in reducing the women's smoking. In fact a comparison between behavioural changes in the intervention and control groups showed differences both in the proportions stopping or reducing and in mean reductions in the daily number of cigarettes smoked (Table 13.2). The greatest behaviour differences were among primiparous women; those in the intervention group were more likely to stop or to reduce their smoking than were the primiparous controls.

**Table 13.2** Changes in smoking behaviour in the intervention and control groups

| Group | $n$ | Type of change (%) | | | | Mean daily reduction of cigarettes |
|---|---|---|---|---|---|---|
| | | Stopped | Reduced | No change | Increased | |
| Intervention | | | | | | |
| Primiparae | 181 | 13 | 34 | 40 | 12 | 3.2 |
| Multiparae | 312 | 7 | 24 | 56 | 13 | 1.6 |
| Total | 493 | 9 | 28 | 50 | 13 | 2.2 |
| Control | | | | | | |
| Primiparae | 197 | 7 | 24 | 53 | 16 | 1.7 |
| Multiparae | 292 | 6 | 17 | 63 | 15 | 0.8 |
| Total | 489 | 6 | 19 | 59 | 16 | 1.1 |

## Infant size at birth

The birth weights, lengths, and head circumferences of the babies were standardized to take account of variation in gestation at delivery, in the sex of the baby, and in maternal height, the latter having differed between intervention and control groups. The standardized differences between the full intervention and control groups were +28 g for birth weight, +0.49 cm for length, and +0.01 cm for head circumference: the difference in length was statistically significant but the differences in weight and head size were not (Table 13.3).

In view of the parity differences between levels of intervention implementation and between subsequent behaviour changes, the outcome differences were then compared among first and later births separately. This showed that the differences in birth weight and length were also concentrated among the primiparous women. The intervention/control difference among first births was +68 g for weight and +0.75 cm for length. The length difference among first births was highly significant and the weight difference now closely approached the 5 per cent level ($P < 0.06$). There was no gestational effect here as mean gestation at delivery in the groups was the same. The systematic correspondence between parity, the quality of advice received, the subsequent response, and the weight and length effects, allow the conclusion that the differences represent a direct effect of anti-smoking intervention upon fetal growth.

## Association between advice and behaviour change

Paradoxically, the incomplete implementation of the anti-smoking intervention supplied additional data that had not been planned. Variations in the

**Table 13.3** Infant size at birth in the intervention and control groups

| Infant size | Intervention ($n = 493$) | Control ($n = 489$) | Standardized difference* | One-tailed $P$† |
|---|---|---|---|---|
| Mean birth weight (g) | | | | |
| Primiparae | 3164 | 3068 | 68 | < 0.06 |
| Multiparae | 3163 | 3171 | −0.5 | 0.50 |
| Total | 3164 | 3130 | 28 | 0.15 |
| Mean length (cm) | | | | |
| Primiparae | 50.69 | 49.88 | 0.75 | < 0.01 |
| Multiparae | 50.67 | 50.31 | 0.29 | 0.13 |
| Total | 50.68 | 50.13 | 0.49 | 0.01 |
| Mean head circumference (cm) | | | | |
| Primiparae | 33.80 | 33.78 | 0.06 | 0.36 |
| Multiparae | 34.00 | 33.97 | 0.04 | 0.35 |
| Total | 33.92 | 33.89 | 0.01 | 0.26 |

* The differences are based upon direct standardization, using gestation, sex of child, and height, of mother.
† A one-tailed test examined the null hypothesis (Ho) that a health education intervention would not improve fetal size. It could be argued *a priori* that health education might be harmful: if this was seriously considered then a two-tailed test would be appropriate. The calculated $P$-values should then be doubled and the findings reinterpreted. Our own preference is for the one-tailed option because all reported non-experimental studies have indicated a negative association between smoking and birth weight, and there is no reported evidence that health education increases smoking. If a two-tailed test was used the acceptability of hypotheses alternative to Ho would be different in the two directions and an asymmetric choice of significance levels called for.

nature of advice received, and differences in the type of staff giving it, allowed comparison between the effects of these implementation differences upon subsequent changes in behaviour. This provides useful supplementary information for guiding health education practice.

The crucial variable with respect to subsequent behaviour change was the content of the advice, rather than the status of the person giving it. Careful advice and information given by a midwife was as effective in improving smoking as the same advice from an obstetrician. The most effective form of intervention was advice to stop smoking completely, accompanied by a discussion about its effects. Of those who received this from the obstetrician, 58 per cent stopped or reduced their smoking, as did 57 per cent of those who received it from the midwife. In these circumstances, the use of the special leaflet had little additional effect. In the absence of verbal advice, however, the leaflet was better than nothing at all. Finally, those women who reported advice only to reduce the number of cigarettes smoked were found to be the group least likely to change: there was indeed *less* improvement in smoking among these women than among those who had neither verbal advice nor the leaflet. Half-hearted advice of this type seemed to have been taken as condoning smoking and great care must be taken in the wording used when discussing with a woman whether she should just cut down.

These additional findings were based on materials not governed by the randomization process so the interpretation is less exact. It is, of course, difficult to be certain whether it was the quality of advice that influenced the women's behaviour: or whether it was the behaviour that resulted in a self-justifying recollection of the advice which she received.

## Discussion

The results of this trial show that a properly planned anti-smoking health education intervention among women having their first baby leads both to altered smoking behaviour and to increased birth weight and birth length of the infants compared with controls. Evidence for multiparous women was inconclusive, mainly because the implementation of the plan was defective. Had the intervention been given exactly as planned to the whole group it might have been possible to influence the multiparae, as well as increasing further the benefit to primiparous women and their infants. These findings offer direct operational guidance for planning the content of antenatal care, but their chief importance is in establishing the causal relationship between smoking and impaired fetal growth.

Two previously reported experiments (Donovan 1977; Sexton and Hebel 1984) used an anti-smoking intervention given by specially designated personnel. This gave the researchers direct control of the intervention, and the hazards of incomplete implementation were thus avoided. However, this approach also incurred a practical disadvantage. The use of a designated 'educator' declares the intent of the study to the women in the intervention group, and identifies them as 'special'. It creates expectations, which might be reflected as much in biased answers to later questions on their smoking behaviour, as in actual behaviour changes. Such design problems might indeed provide an explanation for Donovan's negative results relating to birth weight. The reduced smoking reported by the 'treated' women may not have been real. Donovan did himself consider this possibility, but favoured the alternative explanation that a reduction in smoking after hospital booking was too late to improve fetal growth.

Non-experimental studies of pregnant women who stopped smoking early have shown consistently that the weights of their babies were similar to those of non-smokers (Lowe 1959; Butler *et al.* 1972; Andrews and McGarry 1972; Rantakallio 1978). It has generally been inferred from this that it was only in later pregnancy that smoking retarded fetal growth. Donovan has questioned this inference suggesting instead that women who stop smoking 'on their own' are generally much lighter smokers than those who continue to smoke, and so would also have smoked much less in early pregnancy.

Evidence was sought on these issues from an examination of all the women in this hospital population who had stopped smoking since becoming pregnant, in both the intervention and control groups: and in those who stopped prior to hospital booking (the last group was not included in the randomized experiment). These women were categorized according to the stage of gestation when they had stopped smoking: 85 had stopped before 6 weeks, 119 between 6 and 16 weeks and 56 after 16 weeks. Fetal sizes were calculated for each group and compared with those for non-smokers and for those who continued to smoke throughout pregnancy. For those who stopped before 6 weeks or between 6 and 16 weeks, the birth weights and birth lengths were similar to non-smokers. The 56 women who stopped after 16 weeks had smaller babies than the early stoppers and non-smokers but they were still considerably heavier than among the persistent smokers (MacArthur and Knox 1988). These findings suggest that late stopping still offers a substantial benefit in terms of fetal growth.

However, the question arises again whether these differences are the direct consequence of change in smoking behaviour, or whether they reflect prior social differences. Several studies have shown that women who stop smoking during pregnancy, generally before their contact with hospital antenatal services, differ greatly in their social and demographic characteristics from those who continue to smoke, and in fact resemble non-smokers in these respects (Andrews and McGarry 1972; Baric *et al.* 1976; Donovan 1977; Rush and Cassano 1983). The study of early stoppers reported here has confirmed this. These women will have bigger babies irrespective of the actual withdrawal of tobacco usage. However, the women who stopped smoking later in pregnancy (after 16 weeks) were shown to be different. They were identical to the persistent smokers in their social and demographic characteristics (with the exception of parity), indicating that the differences in fetal size are likely to arise directly from stopping smoking. This group of women is also important in a pragmatic sense. Because they are socially disadvantaged, their infants are exposed to a double hazard. The combined effects of social disadvantage and of smoking-induced low birth weight could be greater than the simple sum of each. There may therefore be a disproportionate benefit to be obtained from changing their smoking behaviour.

The validity of self-reported data must be carefully considered in any study of smoking behaviour. In addition to ensuring that the women were unaware that they were participating in a trial, other precautions were taken to avoid induced bias. In particular great care was taken during the interviews to avoid censorious overtones when asking about smoking. This was the first encounter between the interviewer and the women, and it was made clear that the interviewers were not obstetricians or midwives. Data are routinely collected in the study hospital at antenatal booking on the number of cigarettes currently smoked. Matched with the study data for the same women on level of smoking at the time of booking, it was found that substantially greater numbers of cigarettes had been recorded in the study data. At discharge, after delivery, the women are also asked routinely what had been their average number of cigarettes throughout pregnancy. This was again matched with the study data, with the same result.

Urine specimens were also obtained from a sample of the women in the experiment to seek an objective measure of reported behaviour. Urinary cotinine levels were measured by clinical chemistry colleagues. While this proved capable of distinguishing smokers from non-smokers, the results did not adequately distinguish different levels of smoking. This component of the study was then discontinued.

The USA trial (Sexton and Hebel 1984) produced excellent reductions in smoking, with 27 per cent of the treatment group stopping completely compared with 3 per cent of controls. Correspondingly, this trial obtained a difference of 92 g in weight and 0.6 cm in length. An intensive educational approach was used, conducted in the womens' homes and continuing throughout pregnancy. It incorporated all those health education measures most likely to alter behaviour; support within the social environment could be utilized and the advice tailored specifically to individual requirements. The women were interviewed at the eighth month of pregnancy to avoid any bias from prior knowledge of birth weight, or any birth problems. In addition, an objective biochemical test using salivary thiocyanate was incorporated into the study design, which confirmed the validity of the women's responses.

Sexton and Hebel have since followed-up the children in their sample at age three, to assess the long-term effects of smoking and of stopping smoking during pregnancy. They found differences both in cognitive function and in physical growth among the children of mothers who stopped smoking compared with those who did not (Sexton *et al.* 1990; Fox *et al.* 1990).

A follow-up has just commenced of the children in this Birmingham population, at 9 years of age. Its objectives are to measure the long-term effects of smoking, to see whether intervention and altered behaviour offer benefits in later childhood in terms of physical growth and intelligence, and to measure the degree to which smoking in early pregnancy may have effected irreversible changes.

# References

Andrews, J. and McGarry, J. M. (1972). A community study of smoking in pregnancy. *Journal of Obstetrics and Gynaecology of the British Commonwealth,* **79**, 1057–73.
Baric, L., MacArthur, C., and Sherwood, M. (1976). A study of health education aspects of smoking in pregnancy. *International Journal of Health Education,* **19** (28) (Suppl), 1–17.

Butler, N. R., Goldstein, H., and Ross, E. M. (1972). Cigarette smoking in pregnancy: its influence on birthweight and perinatal mortality. *British Medical Journal*, **ii**, 127–30.

Donovan, J. W. (1977). Randomised controlled trial of anti-smoking advice in pregnancy. *British Journal of Preventive and Social Medicine*, **31**, 6–12.

Fox, N. L., Sexton, M., and Hebel, J. R. (1990). Prenatal exposure to tobacco: effects on physical growth at age three. *International Journal of Epidemiology*, **19**, 66–71.

Lowe, C. (1959). Effect of mother's smoking habits on birthweight of their children. *British Medical Journal*, **iii**, 673–6.

MacArthur, C. and Knox, E. G. (1988). Smoking in pregnancy: effects of stopping at different stages. *British Journal of Obstetrics and Gynaecology*, **95**, 551–5.

MacArthur, C., Newton, J. R., and Knox, E. G. (1987). Effect of anti-smoking health education on infant size at birth: a randomised controlled trial. *British Journal of Obstetrics and Gynaecology*, **94**, 295–300.

Rantakallio, P. (1978). The effect of maternal smoking on birthweight and the subsequent health of the child. *Early Human Development*, **2**, 371–82.

Rush, D. and Cassano, P. (1983). Relationship of cigarette smoking and social class to birthweight and perinatal mortality among all births in Britain. 5–11 April 1970. *Journal of Epidemiology and Community Health*, **37**, 249–55.

Sexton, M. and Hebel, J. R. (1984). A clinical trial of changes in maternal smoking and its effect on birthweight. *Journal of the American Medical Association*, **251**, 911–15.

Sexton, M., Fox, N. L., and Hebel, J. R. (1990). Prenatal exposure to tobacco: effects on cognitive functioning at age three. *International Journal of Epidemiology*, **19**, 72–7.

Surgeon General (1980). *The Health Consequences of Smoking for Women*, pp. 189–239. US Dept Health and Human Sciences. US Government Printing Office.

# 14. Prenatal smoking interventions: programmes with important potential

R Louise Floyd, Carol Hogue, James Marks,
Juliette Kendrick, Christine Zahniser, Eileen Gunter,
and Judy Stevens

## Introduction

Improving pregnancy outcome by providing high-quality prenatal care has been, and continues to be, a major public health priority in the United States. By providing: 'a foundation for improving the health of the pregnant woman, infant, and family,' the prenatal care system: 'is a cornerstone of health care delivery in our society' (US Public Health Service 1989). Prenatal care is the mechanism through which effective screening for risk factors, counselling to reduce risks, and treatment for health conditions is delivered.

Guidelines for content of prenatal care, recently developed by a US Public Health Service expert panel (1989), call for systematic preconception and prenatal counselling to encourage smoking cessation before, during, and after pregnancy. The panel found that: 'among behaviours capable of having adverse effects on pregnancy, smoking has been best studied' (US Public Health Service 1989). The panel judged that scientific evidence is good for an association between maternal smoking and poor pregnancy outcome, for the efficacy of smoking cessation to improve pregnancy outcome, and for the efficacy of health promotion activities that help women stop smoking.

## Scientific evidence

Poor pregnancy outcomes related to maternal smoking include spontaneous abortion, preterm delivery, intra-uterine growth retardation, and sudden infant death syndrome (US Public Health Service 1989; Mullen 1990). Because of the combined effects of preterm delivery and growth retardation, babies of women who smoke throughout pregnancy are twice as likely to weigh less than 2500 g than are babies born to mothers who do not smoke or who quit before or during pregnancy (Niswander and Gordon 1972; Meyer *et al.* 1974; Meyer *et al.* 1976; US Department of Health, Education, and Welfare 1980; Kleinman and Madans 1985; Shiono *et al.* 1986). The risk for low birth weight increases with the amount smoked and is independent of other risk factors for low birth weight (Hogue and Sappenfield 1987).

Maternal smoking increases the risk for perinatal death because smoking decreases birth weight and increases perinatal morbidity independent of birth weight (Kleinman *et al.* 1988; Meyer *et al.* 1976; US Department of Health, Education, and Welfare 1980). Estimates of increased risk range from 1.03 to 1.38 times the risk for children born to non-smokers.

Several prenatal smoking cessation research trials, conducted in the United States and the United Kingdom during the late 1970s and early 1980s, demonstrated that smoking cessation could be enhanced if structured intervention programmes were provided to women during the prenatal period. Among women who were smokers at enrolment, Sexton *et al.* (1987) found a quit rate of 32 per cent for those who participated in intervention activities and only 7 per cent for controls. Other investigators report quit rates ranging from 9 to 22 per cent for women who participated in intervention activities and from 2 to 9 per cent for controls (Windsor *et al.* 1985; Lilley and Forster 1986; MacArthur *et al.* 1987; Ershoff *et al.* 1989). Higher quit rates have been reported for studies that limited interventions to women who entered care early in pregnancy. In addition, some researchers have found that intervention activities contribute to maintenance of cessation for up to 6 months postpartum (Chapter 15).

In the United States, approximately 21 per cent of all pregnant women smoke cigarettes, but the rates of smoking are even higher for women whose risk of having an infant with low birth weight is already high (i.e. the poor, the poorly educated, and teenagers) (Kleinman and Madans 1985; US Department of Health and Human Services 1989; Williamson *et al.* 1989). Although about 15 to 20 per cent of women who smoke quit on their own when they learn they are pregnant, those who do so are generally lighter smokers and better educated than those who continue to smoke (Kleinman and Madans 1985). Thus, an important target population for systematic smoking cessation counselling are less-educated women. The economic costs of smoking during pregnancy are enormous. One study found that babies born to smokers incurred a national total of $267 million (1983 dollars) in neonatal intensive care costs (Oster *et al.* 1988). Another study (Marks *et al.* 1990), which used 1986 dollars and a higher estimate of infants admitted to neonatal intensive care units, estimated the total excess cost at $519 million.

## Programme implementation

In the United States, public health clinics serve low-income clients. Despite sound scientific evidence that maternal smoking increases the risk for poor pregnancy outcome, that quitting smoking after conception reduces such risk, and that structured smoking cessation activities can effectively bring about cessation, systematic cessation counselling is not provided to all pregnant women who smoke and attend publicly funded prenatal care clinics.

In 1989, a survey of state tobacco control activities was conducted by the Association of State and Territorial Health Officers with assistance of the Office on Smoking and Health, Centers for Disease Control (CDC). At the time of the survey, 25 states reported that maternal smoking history was recorded on the birth certificate, but only seven states had analysed the data. One-half of the states surveyed reported that they did not provide cessation activities to women of childbearing age (15–44 years old). Of states that reported activities aimed at this target group, only a few specifically mentioned prenatal smoking cessation programmes. The CDC is in the process of determining more specifically the nature and extent of these activities directed towards women of childbearing age, particularly those who are pregnant.

## Demonstration project

In 1986, the CDC undertook the Smoking Cessation in Pregnancy (SCIP) project to study the application of prenatal smoking cessation technology in broad-based public health clinics that serve mothers and infants. Two states also developed a brief intervention programme for clinics that monitor women's nutritional status and provide food vouchers through the Women, Infants, and Children Food Supplement programme (WIC clinics). The objectives of the SCIP project are:

1. To develop concise smoking cessation interventions to be integrated into these public clinics.
2. To assist low-income pregnant clients to quit smoking.
3. To reduce the rate of low birth weight among low-income women.

The three states chosen to participate in the project are geographically and culturally diverse, and include both rural and urban areas. Colorado, a western, mountainous state, has many Hispanics. Missouri, a mostly rural, mid-western state, has few high-density urban areas. Maryland, on the east coast, has many urban areas and a high percentage of African–Americans.

## Methods

To develop concise smoking cessation interventions to be integrated into these public clinics, the literature, and other existing programmes were thoroughly reviewed. Focus groups were convened consisting of clients in all three states and in one state clinic providers as well. The purpose of these focus groups was to elicit from clients and providers ideas regarding intervention design. One-to-one counselling was chosen as the primary means of conveying cessation information to clients. Because time constraints on clinic staff prohibited extensive counselling, interventions were designed to require no more than 5 to 10 min per session. At the end of the intervention design phase, each of the three states had developed their own unique intervention for prenatal smokers.

## Colorado

The State of Colorado developed seven pamphlets, a 'Mom's Agreement,' and a quit certificate to be used as adjuncts to counselling. These materials are made available in English and Spanish. Colorado's intervention also includes the American Lung Association's flip chart for discussing the health effects of smoking on the fetus, the Los Angeles Lung Association's two-part *Stop smoking and take charge* video (one part is used prenatally and the other postnatally), posters, pin-buttons, and a quit kit. The kit contains cinnamon toothpicks, sunflower seeds, a straw cut in half for inhaling, and other items. A protocol was developed for standardizing the information given to clients at each visit according to their smoking status. Clients are classified as current smokers or recent quitters. During a client's initial visit, a nurse assesses the client's smoking status, discusses health effects on the fetus, sets goals for quitting, discusses quitting methods, and gives the appropriate pamphlets.

An additional intervention is provided to clients of WIC clinics. This 'booster intervention' consists of a 2 min counselling session reinforced by two pamphlets selected from the primary intervention materials. Again, specific activities were outlined for the counsellor to suggest, depending on the client's classification and visit status. Approximately 68 per cent of SCIP clients in Colorado are enrolled in the WIC programme by the eighth month of pregnancy.

## Missouri

The State of Missouri developed six pamphlets for use in conjunction with one-to-one counselling. The hallmark of this programme is a laminated flip chart that discusses six critical areas of smoking cessation:

(1) motivation;
(2) preparation to quit;
(3) the quitting process;
(4) support;
(5) relapse prevention;
(6) hazards of passive smoking.

The Missouri protocol, built around these six areas, includes explicit instructions for the nurse counsellor depending on the client's smoking status and visit status. Refrigerator magnets and a quit kit are also distributed. A booster intervention, provided to WIC programme participants, consists of a 2 min counselling session and two pamphlets specifically designed for this programme. Physicians attending clients in the prenatal clinics are asked to deliver a firm stop smoking message, along with a stop smoking prescription.

## *Maryland*

The State of Maryland developed an intervention consisting of two self-help manuals: *Quit and be free*, which helps smokers quit and *A proud quitter*, which helps quitters maintain non-smoking status. Other materials include an audio tape, refrigerator posters, a quit kit, and an infant T-shirt. Providers use a five-step approach to counselling clients:

(1) assessment;
(2) problem-solving;
(3) advice;
(4) making a contract;
(5) follow-up.

Protocols address three types of clients: women who want to quit, women who don't want to quit, and women who have quit. Each counselling session follows the five-step approach, and clients are guided in the use of the self-help manuals.

## Research design

The three intervention strategies are being tested through a carefully designed quasi-experimental study. Public clinics in each of the three states were randomly assigned to intervention and control groups. All smokers who attended the intervention clinics during the intake period were eligible for the study. A smoker was defined as anyone who had smoked, even a puff, in the last 7 days, or who had smoked in the 7 days before she thought she was pregnant (even if she had since quit). For the latter group of women, the intention is to help them maintain their quit status during pregnancy. Training sessions were conducted at all sites to provide instructions for data collection and data management. Special training sessions were conducted at intervention sites to familiarize the clinic staff with the intervention and its use. Approximately 140 sites (including prenatal and WIC clinics) are involved in the study, and are in the final stages of data collection.

The interventions will be evaluated by using both process and outcome measures. Process instruments include monthly telephone checklists, quarterly site visit reports, client opinion forms, prenatal provider opinion forms, and WIC provider opinion forms. Outcome data are gathered from questionnaires completed at the initial, 8-month, and postpartum visits. These data include medical history and information about stress, smoking status, caffeine and alcohol consumption, prenatal care, and outcome of delivery. A client's self-reported smoking status will be validated by using urine cotinine measurements.

Preliminary results are now available from Colorado and Missouri. Using self-reported data only, it appeared that clients attending the intervention clinics were 50 per cent more likely to quit smoking than were those attending the control clinics. When self-reported smoking status was validated with urine cotinine, there was 90 per cent overall agreement between the two. However, among the self-reported nonsmokers at enrolment, 21 per cent in Colorado and 36 per cent in Missouri had cotinine values consistent with active smoking (nondisclosure). After correcting for nondisclosure, there was no difference in cessation at the eighth month among those in the intervention group versus those in the control group (Kendrick *et al.* 1991). Maryland data are pending, and further analyses of existing data are underway. However, it is clear from current data that nondisclosure is a key issue in prenatal smoking cessation for both research and programme dissemination.

Preliminary results from process evaluation efforts indicate that programmes like the one in Colorado can be successfully integrated into public prenatal and WIC clinics. Anonymous client opinion forms collected at the post-partum visit from the first 97 women who received the intervention were reviewed. Forty-six per cent of respondents reported that they had quit smoking for 7 or more days, at an average of 3.1 attempts; 82 per cent reported that they cut down by at least half. Eighty-seven per cent said that they had read all or some of the brochures; 56 per cent found them helpful or very helpful. When clients were asked how helpful the various components of the intervention were in helping them to quit or cut down, it was found that talking with the nurse was rated as helpful or very helpful by 68 per cent. Learning about coping with urges to smoke (44 per cent), receiving instructions on quitting tips (44 per cent), and having a buddy (43 per cent) received the next highest number of responses. Setting a date to quit smoking was reported as helpful or very helpful by only 16 per cent of respondents. The client opinion form was also offered to women in the control clinics. Of the first 79 respondents, 55 per cent reported having read some pamphlets, and 56 per cent reported that talking with the nurse was helpful or very helpful. Among those women in control clinics who responded to the opinion form, 34 per cent reported that they quit smoking for 7 or more days with an average of 2.2 attempts, and 74 per cent reported that they had cut down by at least half.

Although these results are preliminary, they do permit a few tentative postulates. First, many respondents to the client opinion form at both inter-vention and control clinics tried to quit smoking at some point(s) during pregnancy. It is not known if those who did not attempt to quit were positively affected by any of the interventions. Second, women in the control clinics were receiving some stop smoking messages. This is not surprising, as Colorado has a history of strong health promotion activities in their prenatal care clinics. It may also explain the relatively high rate of cessation found among controls in this trial, as compared with controls of other trials (e.g. Windsor *et al.* 1985). Third, the high percentage of women who reported that contact with the nurse was helpful supports the assumption based on the literature that the one-to-one approach is important to achieving cessation.

In Colorado, providers of the new intervention were surveyed after data collection was completed. They reported spending between 2 and 10 min on the initial visit and 1–5 min on subsequent visits. They believed that the training had been adequate, and they were comfortable with their ability to use the new techniques with patients. The most frequently cited major obstacle was patient's perceived lack of interest.

## Cost-effectiveness of structured smoking cessation programmes

To be accepted as a routine component of prenatal care, structured smoking cessation counselling must be cost-effective. Doubilet's definition of a cost-effective programme is one that will: 'improve health outcome and save money or deliver a health benefit at an acceptable cost' (Doubilet *et al*. 1983). In another study, Marks and colleagues (1990) estimated the cost-effectiveness of a smoking cessation programme for pregnant women designed to reduce low birth weight and perinatal mortality. The hypothetical programme would consist of a single 15-min counselling session, printed materials (at $5 per patient), and two follow-up telephone calls for an estimated 30 min of staff time (nurse or health educator) for each call. The total programme cost would be $30 per participant (including overheads and staff training). The health impact of such a programme was estimated by using the following assumptions: 21 per cent of pregnant women smoke; 15 per cent of smokers would quit if offered structured counselling and their risk for having a low birth weight infant (10 per cent) would become that of non-smokers (5 per cent); and risk for perinatal mortality would be decreased by 20 per cent among smokers who quit as a result of the programme.

Under these assumptions, it would cost $4000 for every infant whose birth weight was raised from low to normal. The savings, from preventing costly hospitalizations for low birth weight infants and long-term care for infants who survive badly handicapped, were estimated at more than $6 for every $1 spent on a smoking cessation programme. These figures compare favourably with an estimate of $3.4 saved per $1 spent on prenatal care (Institute of Medicine 1985).

The cost per infant death prevented was estimated at $69 542 (1986 dollars), or $2934 for each year of life gained (assuming a life expectancy of 75 years, discounted at 4 per cent). These estimates are roughly comparable with those found for improving survival of very low birth weight infants (1000–1499 g) through neonatal intensive care—$52 000 (1978 dollars) per survivor and $2540 per year of life gained (Boyle *et al*. 1983).

Prenatal programmes working with women at high risk of low birth weight due to other causes (e.g. young age, low education, etc.) might find lower quit rates or might need more intensive, higher-cost interventions than assumed in the cost-effectiveness study. Yet, the prevalence of low birth weight is greater in these high-risk populations. Because the number of low birth weight births prevented is a function of prevalence of low birthweight and the quit rate, among a higher-risk group that has twice the underlying risk of low birth weight the quit rate could be one-half as great as that for the lower-risk group, and the same number of low birth weight births would be prevented. Alternatively, if the same number of women quit in the higher-risk group as in the lower-risk group, the greater benefit would tend to offset the greater costs of the programme required to provide interventions to high risk groups. However, one study conducted in a high risk population found very low costs/quitter using a self-help programme (Windsor *et al.* 1988).

## Conclusion

Systematic smoking cessation counselling has not yet been introduced into most public prenatal care practices in the United States. As a result, little of the morbidity and mortality associated with smoking during pregnancy is being prevented. The US Public Health Service has a commitment to increase the availability of such programmes to public health users whose prevalence of smoking is often higher than that found in the general population. Through such programmes, it is estimated that several thousand low birth weight births could be prevented and several hundred lives saved each year, at an estimated cost savings of $6 per $1 spent on the programme.

## References

Boyle, M. H., Torrance, G. W., Sinclair, J. C., and Horwood, S. P. (1983). Economic evaluation of neonatal intensive care of very low birth-weight infants. *New England Journal of Medicine*, **308**, 1330–7.

Doubilet, P., Weinstein, M. C., and McNeil, B. J. (1983). Use and misuse of the term 'cost effective' in medicine. *New England Journal of Medicine*, **314**, 253–6.

Ershoff, D. H., Mullen, P. D., and Quinn, V. P. (1989). A randomised trial of a serialised self-help smoking cessation program for pregnant women in an HMO. *American Journal of Public Health*, **79**, 182–7.

Hogue, C. J. R. and Sappenfield, W. (1987). Smoking and low birth weight. Current concepts. In *Smoking and reproductive health*, (ed. M. Rosenberg), pp. 97–103. PSG, Littleton, Massachusetts.

Institute of Medicine. (1985). *Preventing low birthweight*. National Academy Press. Washington DC.

Kendrick, J. S., Zahniser, S. C., Floyd, R. L., Gargiullo, P. M., Salas, N. M., Miller, N., Spierto, F. W., Metzger, R., and Stockbauer, J. (1991). *Nondisclosure of smoking status in intervention programs for public prenatal clients*. Poster session, 1991 Annual Meeting of the American Public Health Association, Atlanta, Georgia.

Kleinman, J. C. and Madans, J. H. (1985). The effects of maternal smoking, physical stature, and educational attainment on the incidence of low birth weight. *American Journal of Epidemiology*, **121**, 843–5.

Kleinman, J. C., Pierre, M. B., Madans, J. H., Land, G. H., and Schramm, W. F. (1988). The effects of maternal smoking on fetal and infant mortality. *American Journal of Epidemiology*, **27**, 274–82.

Lilley, J. and Forster, D. P. (1986). A randomized controlled trial of individual counselling of smokers in pregnancy. *Public Health Reports*, **100**, 309–15.

MacArthur, C., Newton, J. R., and Knox, E. G. (1987). Effect of antismoking health education on infant size at birth: A randomized controlled trial. *British Journal of Obstetrics and Gynaecology*, **94**, 295–300.

Marks, J. S., Koplan, J. P., Hogue, C. J. R., and Dalmat, M. E. (1990). A cost-benefit/cost-effectiveness analysis of smoking cessation for pregnant women. *American Journal of Preventive Medicine*, **6(5)**, 282–9.

Meyer, M. B., Tonascia, J. T., and Buck, C. (1974). The interrelationship of maternal smoking and increased perinatal mortality with other risk factors. Further analysis of the Ontario Perinatal Mortality Study, 1960–1961. *American Journal of Epidemiology*, **100**, 443–52.

Meyer, M. B., Jonas, B. S., and Tonascia, J. T. (1976). Perinatal events associated with maternal smoking during pregnancy. *American Journal of Epidemiology*, **103**, 464–76.

Mullen, Patricia D. (1990). Smoking cessation counseling in prenatal care. In *New perspectives on prenatal care*, (ed. I. R. Merkatz and J. E. Thompson), pp. 161–76. Elsevier Science Publishing Co., Inc., New York.

Niswander, K. R. and Gordon, M. (eds.) (1972). *The women and their pregnancies*. W. B. Saunders Co., Philadelphia.

Oster, G., Delea, T. E., and Colditz, G. A. (1988). Maternal smoking during pregnancy and expenditures on neonatal health care. *American Journal of Preventive Medicine*, **4**, 216–19.

Sexton, M., Hebel, J. R., and Fox, N. L. (1987). Postpartum smoking. In *Smoking and reproduction*, (ed. M. J. Rosenberg), pp. 222–6. PSG-Yearbook, Littleton, Massachusetts.

Shiono, P. H., Klebanoff, M. A., and Rhoads, G. G. (1986). Smoking and drinking during pregnancy: their effects on preterm birth. *Journal of the American Medical Association*, **255**, 82–4.

US Department of Health, Education and Welfare (1980). *The health consequences of smoking for women: a report of the Surgeon General*. U.S. Department of Health, Education and Welfare, Public Health Service, Office on Smoking and Health, Washington DC.

US Department of Health and Human Services (1989). *Reducing the health consequences of smoking: 25 years of progress. A report of the Surgeon General*, DHHS publication No. (CDC) 89-8411. U.S. Department of Health and Human Services, Public Health Service, Centers for Disease Control, Center for Chronic Disease Prevention and Health Promotion, Office on Smoking and Health. Washington DC.

US Public Health Service (1989). *Caring for our future: the content of prenatal care*. A report of the Public Health Service Expert Panel on Content of Prenatal Care. U.S. Public Health Service, Washington DC.

Williamson, D. F., Serdula, M. K., Kendrick, J. S., and Binkin, N. J. (1989). Comparing the prevalence of smoking in pregnant and non-pregnant women, 1985 to 1986. *Journal of the American Medical Association*, **261**, 70–4.

Windsor, R. A., Cutter, G., Morris, J., *et al.* (1985). The effectiveness of smoking cessation methods for smokers in public health maternity clinics: a randomized trial. *American Journal of Reproductive Health*, **75**, 1389–92.

Windsor, R. A., Warner, K. E., and Cutter, G. R. (1988). A cost-effectiveness analysis of self-help smoking cessation methods for pregnant women. *Public Health Reports*, **103**, 83–8.

# 15. Anti-smoking intervention during pregnancy: impact on smoking behaviour and birth weight

*Pamela Gillies*

## Introduction

The associations between maternal smoking, low birth weight babies and perinatal morbidity and mortality are well established (Royal College of Physicians 1977), as are the risks of smoking to the mothers' own health (Doll *et al.* 1980). In view of the smoking-related health hazards for women and their babies, it is surprising that relatively few attempts have been made in industrialized countries to provide women with additional help to give up smoking during pregnancy and evaluate the effectiveness of intervention (Windsor and Orleans 1986).

The findings from recent randomized controlled trials of anti-smoking interventions in the UK (Donovan 1977; MacArthur *et al.* 1987) and USA (Sexton and Hebel 1984; Windsor *et al.* 1985; Simmons 1988), which had relatively large sample populations are summarized in Table 15.1. On balance, the evidence indicates that anti-smoking intervention in pregnancy is likely to have a positive impact on levels of tobacco consumption and can, in the USA, also affect smoking cessation rates. The evidence pertaining to the impact of intervention on smoking and thereby on birth weight is, however, equivocal. Simmons' (1988) study of low income women in the USA found no effect of anti-smoking intervention on smoking or birth weight. Donovan (1977) in the UK found decreased tobacco consumption levels but no impact on birth weight, whilst MacArthur *et al.* (1987) noted decreased consumption levels and a slight, though not statistically significant, effect on birth weight in first-born babies only. Sexton and Hebel (1984) found an impact on smoking behaviour and a significantly higher birth weight in babies born to women in their intervention group.

The main aim of the study described in this paper was to record the impact of an anti-smoking project based in an antenatal clinic on smoking cessation and reinforcement of non-smoking early in pregnancy, in the short-term up to delivery, and in the longer-term up to 6 months after delivery. Only one previous study (Simmons 1988) has attempted long-term evaluation of the impact of intervention on women's smoking. Given the equivocal nature of the findings regarding the relationship between increased birth weight, smok-

**Table 15.1** Randomized controlled trials of anti-smoking interventions in pregnancy and their effect on women's smoking and their babies' birth weight

| Author | Year reported and place | Type of intervention | Outcome | |
|---|---|---|---|---|
| | | | Women's smoking | Birth weight |
| Donovan | 1977 London, UK | Advice by doctor at each antenatal visit | Decreased consumption | No effect |
| Sexton and Hebel | 1984 Baltimore, USA | Home visit, advice, phone call, mail | Increased cessation Decreased consumption | Significantly heavier in experimental group ($P < 0.05$) |
| Windsor *et al.* | 1985 Birmingham, Alabama, USA | Counselling, booklet, self-help guide | Increased cessation Decreased consumption | Not recorded |
| MacArthur *et al.* | 1987 Birmingham, UK | Advice by obstetrician and leaflet | Decreased consumption | An effect on first-born babies only ($P < 0.06$) |
| Simmons | 1988 Los Angeles, USA | Counselling, booklet, bib, postcard, certificate, slide cassette | No effect | No effect |

ing cessation, and health education intervention, this study also aimed to assess the effect of the project in terms of babies' birth weight. The project emphasized the importance of women giving up for their own sake as well as for the good of their babies.

The intervention involved counselling, specially prepared booklets, and the use of a carbon monoxide monitor in a busy antenatal clinic. The health education approach adopted involved changes to the environment of the clinic and additions to available resources in terms of both equipment and midwifery staffing. This approach did not allow the randomization of women into experimental and control groups and necessitated a matched control design where antenatal clinics were matched. Whilst this design is not as powerful as a randomized trial, the findings can contribute to the body of knowledge pertaining to the impact of intervention, not only on women's smoking but on the impact of changes in smoking during pregnancy upon 'clinical' outcomes such as birth weight.

# Methods

## Sample

All new antenatal clinic attenders at Nottingham's University and City Hospitals who indicated that they smoked or had stopped smoking since they knew they were pregnant and who were less than 32 weeks pregnant, were enrolled in the study. A question on smoking history is a standard part of both hospitals' booking procedure at first antenatal clinic attendance. The sample included 'recent quitters' (women who stopped smoking since learning they were pregnant and before presenting at the antenatal clinic) in addition to current smokers at booking in the antenatal clinic in order to test the impact of the intervention on rates of relapse.

## Study design and data collection

Data were collected by confidential self-completed questionnaires completed by women in both experimental and control clinics at their first antenatal visit, postnatally whilst still in hospital, and 6 months later by post. Response to the 6-month postal questionnaire was encouraged by two reminder letters. In addition to questionnaire responses, a 10 per cent random sample of experimental women ($n = 49$) was interviewed by the researcher whilst still in hospital after the birth.

Amongst other items, the questionnaires asked for information about smoking and changes in smoking behaviour, intentions regarding smoking behaviour, partners' smoking, reasons for smoking, and occupation. Data on birth weights were obtained from obstetric records.

*Reliability* The reliability of women's response to questions about smoking was assessed in the 10 per cent sample by comparing smoking behaviour reported in the postnatal questionnaire with that reported by the same women at the postnatal interview.

*Validity of data* During the course of the project, the project facilitator studied 254 women in the antenatal clinic (54 per cent of the experimental group) using the carbon monoxide (CO) monitor, which was designed by the author. Actual CO levels were recorded and matched with self-reported smoking history given on completed questionnaires. The women observed comprised an 'opportunity' sample.

## The intervention

This comprised four elements:

1. A facilitator was available to answer queries and provide friendly advice and encouragement at first booking and at subsequent antenatal visits. The

initial plan was to train and use a midwife in the clinic to provide this encouragement and help. Lack of staff able to take on this role necessitated the introduction of a researcher in the capacity of 'designated midwife'. The 'friendly encourager', face-to-face counselling approach is recognized to be one of the most effective means of health education (Russell *et al.* 1979; Tones 1986).

2. The programme made available in the clinic a CO monitor designed by the author for women to use to check and record their own progress in stopping or giving up smoking. The use of such monitors in a general practice context has been shown to significantly enhance the effect of verbal advice given to patients to help them stop smoking (Jamrozik *et al.* 1984).

3. The women were offered a specially written book about the project, about the immediate physiological effects of smoking and how it was as important for women to give up smoking for themselves as for their babies. The booklet was designed to be easy to read, as the baseline study (Madeley *et al.* 1989) had shown that women who smoked tended to be younger and to have left school earlier than women who did not smoke.

4. In view of the findings from previous research, which suggested that health education in pregnancy should be more personalized (Windsor *et al.* 1985), mothers were offered the opportunity to attend self-help groups in the hospital.

## Costing the project

Details of the resource input costs of the project, including facilitator's salary, carbon monoxide monitor and associated tubes and cleaning fluid, and printing of booklets were recorded. Indirect or 'hidden' project costs, such as clerical staff time, other midwifery staff time and so on, were not costed in financial terms.

## Analysis

Data were analysed using the SPSSX computer programme. Chi-square tests and *t*-tests were applied where appropriate. A one-tailed *t*-test was used to test the null hypothesis that the health education intervention would not increase fetal birth weight. This approach, suggested by MacArthur *et al.* (1987), was adopted for the following reasons:

1. All the reported evidence suggests that smoking is associated with decreased birthweight.
2. There is no evidence to support the view that health education increases smoking in pregnant women.
3. There is evidence that health education reduces the proportion of women who increase their level of tobacco consumption during pregnancy.

# Results

## Initial response

Between January and June 1987, 498 women at the experimental hospital (University) and 680 at the control hospital (City) were enrolled. Of those enrolled, 475 (95 per cent) of those at the experimental clinic satisfactorily completed a questionnaire about their smoking habits during their first clinic visit. In the control clinic 409 (60 per cent) of those enrolled completed the first questionnaire. The poor level of initial response of the eligible control population does give cause for concern. However, a comparison between the experimental and control group at pretesting had provided strong evidence to support the view that the groups were still comparable for the key variables given in Table 15.2.

## Follow-up response to questionnaire

Of women who completed the initial questionnaire, 25 (5 per cent) from University Hospital (experimental) and 18 (4 per cent) from the City Hospital (control) were lost to the study sample (Table 15.3). Nine left the area during their pregnancy; five were excluded due to having stillborn babies or perinatal deaths; 26 were excluded after spontaneous abortion or termination; one was found not to be pregnant; one baby was put up for adoption and the pregnancy was excluded; and one was found to have stopped smoking before pregnancy. Participation with the postnatal questionnaire amongst the remainder was high, at 85 per cent overall. No differences were recorded between experimental and control groups postnatally in relation to social class, smoking history, or smoking intentions, in those who completed both questionnaires. Comparability of groups in important respects at follow-up was therefore maintained despite further attrition.

## Reliability and validity of response

*Reliability*  Data from questionnaire and interview methods were available for 49 women and an extremely high level of agreement was recorded. Only one of the women who claimed a reduction in consumption, 'changed' her response to 'smoking the same' at interview.

*Validity*  An indication of validity of self-completed smoking history was gained from the 'opportunity' sample studied. Of 206 women who reported themselves as smokers on the questionnaire, all (100 per cent) had carbon monoxide levels above the cut-off point of 10 parts per million (p.p.m.) for detecting smokers. Of 48 women observed who reported having stopped smoking before or after their first antenatal visit, only 1 (2 per cent) registered above 10 p.p.m. on the carbon monoxide monitor.

**Table 15.2** Comparability of experimental and control groups at preproject testing

| Variable | Group | | | |
|---|---|---|---|---|
| | Experimental | | Control | |
| | *n* | % | *n* | % |
| SOCIAL CLASS: (partner's occupation) | | | | |
| Non-manual I | 6 | 2 | 3 | 1 |
| Non-manual II | 48 | 13 | 30 | 10 |
| Non-manual IIIa | 42 | 12 | 26 | 9 |
| Manual IIIb | 158 | 43 | 130 | 43 |
| Manual IV | 74 | 20 | 73 | 24 |
| Manual V | 36 | 10 | 42 | 14 |
| $\chi^2 = 6.8$; df = 5; Not Significant | | | | |
| Own smoking | | | | |
| Daily | 352 | 91 | 344 | 91 |
| Occasionally | 35 | 9 | 34 | 9 |
| $\chi^2 = 0.0$; df = 1; Not Significant | | | | |
| Live with a partner who smokes | | | | |
| Yes | 314 | 67 | 285 | 71 |
| No | 160 | 33 | 117 | 29 |
| $\chi^2 = 2.0$; df = 1; Not Significant | | | | |
| Marital status | | | | |
| Married | 209 | 44 | 189 | 46 |
| Divorced/separated | 23 | 5 | 28 | 7 |
| Single | 96 | 20 | 98 | 24 |
| Living with partner | 142 | 31 | 93 | 23 |
| $\chi^2 = 7.4$; df = 3; Not Significant | | | | |
| Education | | | | |
| Left school < 16 yrs | 356 | 78 | 333 | 83 |
| Left school > 17 yrs | 99 | 22 | 67 | 17 |
| $\chi^2 = 3.1$; df = 1: Not Significant | | | | |
| Age (years) | Mean = 24.5 | | Mean = 24.6 | |
| | SD = 5.158 | | SD = 5.378 | |
| | *n* = 474 | | *n* = 407 | |
| | $t = 0.04$; df = 879; Not Significant | | | |

**Table 15.3** Questionnaire response

| | Completion of first questionnaire in antenatal clinic at first visit (n) | Mothers* completing delivery at University or City Hospital (n) | Completion of questionnaire post-birth in hospital | | Completion of questionnaire 6 months after birth, by post | |
|---|---|---|---|---|---|---|
| | | | (n) | % of those who completed delivery at experimental or control hospitals | (n) | % of those who completed delivery at experimental or control hospitals |
| University Hospital (experimental) | 475 | 450 | 419 | 93 | 236 | 52 |
| City Hospital (control) | 409 | 391 | 296 | 76 | 172 | 44 |

* After exclusions for stillbirths, spontaneous abortions, women who left the area during pregnancy, etc. but including twins

## Participation in all aspects of the project

All women enrolled in the project had a face-to-face counselling session with the project facilitator at least twice before giving birth. All women enrolled in the project received a booklet. The carbon monoxide monitor was used over 1000 times during the project, equivalent to more than twice per woman. Monitor use was, however, voluntary and one woman may have used the machine a number of times whilst another may have decided against use. The option of attending self-help groups was not, however, taken up by any of the women in the study due, amongst other things, to difficulties in returning to the hospital for sessions additional to clinic attendance. This was therefore abandoned. Of the 419 experimental group women who completed a post-natal questionnaire in hospital 418 (99.8 per cent) said they remembered the project and were able to describe it and to give their personal reactions to it (Power *et al.* 1989).

## Changes in smoking behaviour

Table 15.4 shows that significantly more of the experimental than the control women had stopped smoking immediately after birth and 6 months later. The intervention had its greatest effect on maintaining the non-smoking status of women who had stopped smoking before attending the antenatal clinic. Twenty per cent (83/419) of the experimental group and 17 per cent (49/296) of the controls who completed ante- and postnatal questionnaires were identified as having stopped smoking since they first knew they were pregnant and before coming to the antenatal clinic. Significantly, more of these 'early quitters' in the experimental group, 77 per cent (64/83), were still non-smokers immediately after birth when compared with 'early quitters' in the control group 29 per cent (14/49) ($\chi^2 = 28.1$; df = 10 $P < 0.001$). Mothers who participated in the project were more likely than those who did not to have stopped smoking between the time of their first antenatal visit up to the postnatal period, 27/336 compared with 14/247, although the difference did not reach statistical significance.

## Birth weights

There were no differences between groups in the mean weight of babies at birth. The mean birth weight of the babies of the 440 women in the experimental group who were enrolled in the project and who delivered at the University Hospital was 3.19 kg. This was not significantly different from the mean birth weight of 3.16 kg of 390 babies of control women and born in the City Hospital (Table 15.5). In the experimental group, 9 per cent (42/440) babies weighed under 2.5 kg at birth compared with 8 per cent (30/390) in the control group ($\chi^2 = 0.7$; df = 1; not significant). The mean birth weight of the babies weighing under 2.5 kg in the experimental group was not significantly greater than the mean for corresponding babies in the control group (Table 15.5).

**Table 15.4** Women who stopped smoking during pregnancy and who remained non-smokers postbirth

| Group | Stopped smoking since pregnant and still stopped at delivery | | Smoking at delivery | |
|---|---|---|---|---|
| | $n$ | % | $n$ | % |
| Experimental ($n = 419$) | 91 | 22 | 328 | 78 |
| Control ($n = 296$) | 28 | 9 | 268 | 91 |
| Chi-square test | $\chi^2 = 17.9$; df = 1; $P < 0.001$ | | | |

| Group | Stopped smoking since pregnant and still stopped 6 months after delivery | | Smoking 6 months after delivery | |
|---|---|---|---|---|
| | $n$ | % | $n$ | % |
| Experimental ($n = 236$) | 43 | 18 | 193 | 72 |
| Control ($n = 172$) | 19 | 11 | 153 | 89 |
| | $\chi^2 = 3.97$; df = 1; $P < 0.05$ | | | |

**Table 15.5** Mean birth weights by group for all babies and those < 2.5 kg

| Babies | Group | n cases | Mean (kg) | Standard deviation | t value | Degrees freedom | 1-tailed probability | Significance |
|---|---|---|---|---|---|---|---|---|
| All | Experimental* | 440 | 3.191 | 0.542 | 0.90 | 829 | 0.184 | NS |
|  | Control† | 390 | 3.158 | 0.507 |  |  |  |  |
| <2.5 kg | Experimental | 42 | 2.111 | 0.337 | 0.37 | 70 | 0.355 | NS |
|  | Control | 30 | 2.078 | 0.400 |  |  |  |  |

* Missing value in 10 cases.
† Missing value in 1 case.
NS, not significant.

## 'Crude' economic costs of the project

The financial cost of the project for 1 year, including the salary of the facilitator, carbon monoxide monitor, and booklets was £16 936 sterling. At delivery, 13 per cent more experimental than control women had stopped smoking or remained non-smokers since early in pregnancy, equivalent to 55 of the 419 'experimental' group who had responded after birth. The 'raw' or 'crude' financial cost to stop one woman in the intervention group smoking up to delivery was therefore £16 936/55 = £308.

By the 6-month follow-up, 7 per cent more experimental than control women were still non-smokers, equivalent to 17 of the 236 in the intervention group who responded postbirth. The crude cost to stop one woman in the intervention group smoking during pregnancy and for up to 6 months thereafter was £16 936/17 = £996.

## Discussion

### Smoking behaviour

Randomized trials of interventions in the UK have demonstrated that advice and booklets can reduce tobacco consumption in women during pregnancy, but have failed to influence overall rates of smoking cessation (Donovan 1977; MacArthur *et al.* 1987). A very recent small matched trial of the impact of increased advice during pregnancy from community midwives in Southampton found a significant difference between experimental and control groups when smoking cessation and reduction in consumption levels were combined (Shakespeare and Batten 1990). The findings of the study reported here suggest that intervention can have a significant impact on reinforcing non-smoking and reducing levels of tobacco consumption in women up to and beyond birth. The effectiveness of this study may relate to the fact that, like interventions in the USA, particular efforts were made to personalize the anti-smoking advice given and to offer friendly support and encouragement to women. As in the community midwife counselling study in Southampton (Shakespeare and Batten 1990) the support provided in the Nottingham Mothers Stop Smoking Project focused on the anticipated benefits to women themselves from giving up the smoking habit, and on alternative coping strategies. It did not dwell upon the harm that smoking may do to the unborn baby or on the effect passive smoking may have on the respiratory health of newly born infants.

The attempt to further personalize the intervention by providing the option of self-help groups in the hospital foundered. Women explained that their lack of interest in self-help groups was mainly due to the practical difficulties they would face in returning to the hospital for sessions additional to clinic attendance. Windsor *et al.* (1985) reported a similar experience in the USA, where attempts to bring pregnant smokers together for peer-led discussion on cessation failed due to organizational difficulties. In an Australian study (Ryan *et al.* 1980), pregnant women failed to attend similar groups for a variety of reasons, ranging from not seeing the need, responsibilities to their children, and transport problems.

The relative success of this project may in part be due to the fact that the sample included those who had given up early in pregnancy. Recidivism in those who stop smoking early in pregnancy is high, with over half of the women who stop early in pregnancy re-starting during pregnancy (Gillies *et al.* 1987), and it was felt important to offer reinforcement to these women. This approach appears to have been justified in that the project had its greatest impact on reinforcing non-smoking in women who gave up the habit when they first knew they were pregnant, or early in pregnancy, before attending an antenatal clinic. The significant impact of the project persisted for up to 6 months after delivery. The findings from the long-term follow-up must, however, be interpreted with caution, as only half of the women in experimental and control groups responded at the follow-up stage. The only other long-term follow-up of intervention during pregnancy was carried out in the USA and had only a 1 in 4 response at 6-month follow-up. No effect of intervention on smoking was found in low income women in either the short- or longer-term (Simmons 1988).

## Methodological considerations

An important methodological issue to be considered in assessing the findings presented here is that this present study had a matched case-control rather than a randomized design. Demographic data from a baseline survey of 3483 pregnant women attending the experimental and control antenatal clinics used in this intervention study and undertaken just prior to this study, found no statistically significant differences in the proportion of women attending the antenatal clinics of the University or City Hospitals with regard to marital status (married 72 and 71 per cent, respectively; divorced/separated 3 and 3 per cent; single 12 and 13.7 per cent and living with a partner 13 and 12 per cent respectively); education (percentage who left school under or at 16 years of age, 67 and 69 per cent, respectively); age of women (mean age = 26.05 and 26.33, respectively); social class (I, II and IIINM: 39 and 35 per cent; IIIM: 37 and 41 per cent; IV: 18 and 17 per cent; V: 6 and 6 per cent); proportion with partners unemployed (4 and 3.6 per cent); suburban as opposed to inner city dwellers (64 and 59 per cent); number of times attended hospital during pregnancy (4.8 times and 4.1 times) and smoking (30 per cent smokers at each hospital) (Madeley *et al.* 1989). In addition, a study by Windsor-Richards and Gillies (1988) carried out at the same time as this controlled trial, found no differences between the women giving birth in the two hospitals with regard to ethnic mix, rates of induction and acceleration, fetal monitoring, or type of delivery. These studies established that the populations of women attending the two clinics were comparable on key socio-demographic, obstetric, and behavioural variables and were therefore suitable for participation in a matched controlled trial. Of all births in Nottingham, 99 per cent take place in hospital (Trent Regional Health Authority 1984).

Comparison of experimental and control groups at pretesting of the questionnaires also provided strong evidence to support the view that the groups were comparable on important variables (see Table 15.2). However, it must be borne in mind that the initial response rate in the control group was only 60 per cent, probably because a new member of the midwifery staff was not informed of the project and failed to distribute the questionnaire at a series of clinics. This problem was unanticipated due to the relatively successful running of the baseline survey carried out 9 months prior to this investigation.

It could be argued that the impact of the project may simply have reflected differing inputs in ongoing health education from obstetricians. Obstetricians were not asked to alter their routine health education advice to smoking women in either hospital. At the time of this study, one professor oversaw the medical staffing and input of the antenatal clinics. There is no evidence to suggest that the routine advice given by obstetricians differed markedly during the study time period. No new members of medical staff were recruited in either hospital during the study. In addition, it should be noted that the baseline survey carried out prior to the intervention showed that only one-third of women who smoked in both hospitals remembered receiving advice about their smoking from the obstetrician (Madeley *et al.* 1989).

One final issue to be considered when comparing the findings from study groups relates to the potential impact of the facilitator on women's self-reported smoking. Given that women in this study tended to form a relationship with the facilitator/midwife counsellor, it is feasible that this may have biased their self-reported smoking levels. They may have been more reluctant than controls to report their 'true' smoking status. The limited evidence available in this study from an 'opportunity sample', whose carbon monoxide levels in expired air were compared with self-reported smoking, suggests that only 2 per cent of women failed to provide accurate reports of their smoking status. Windsor *et al.* (1985) reported a similarly low false-positive rate of 3 per cent in a US study where salivary thiocyanate was used as an objective measure of self-reported smoking in pregnant women in an intervention study, tested just prior to giving birth.

## Birth weight

Whilst the main aim of the study reported here was to observe the impact of intervention on women's smoking, the availability of an 'outcome' indicator, such as babies' birth weight at delivery, coupled with the association between low birth weight and perinatal mortality, made it not only feasible but also important to describe the relationship between smoking cessation and birth weight. Only one randomized controlled trial in the USA (Sexton and Hebel 1984) has demonstrated a relationship between increased cessation during pregnancy, decreased consumption, and a significantly higher birth weight in babies born to experimental women. Two further large USA studies, one undertaken across the USA by the Centres for Disease Control (Floyd *et al.* 1990) and one randomized controlled trial of an intervention to prevent relapse in smoking cessation during pregnancy (Lowe *et al.* 1990) have reported preliminary data that suggest increases in smoking cessation rates but no differences between experimental and control groups in birth weight at delivery.

The study reported here found no statistically significant impact of intervention on birth weight, although there was a 33 g difference in mean birth weight recorded between the experimental and control groups, and the project did reinforce cessation. It could be that sample size in many studies evaluating interventions have simply not been large enough to detect a significant impact on birth weight.

One UK study to report an effect of intervention on birth weight, but in first-born babies only, was that of MacArthur *et al.* (1987). Their intervention had reduced consumption and this was reflected in a difference in birth weight between experimental and control babies, but overall this difference did not quite reach statistical significance. The relevance of all the UK findings on birth weight should perhaps be placed in context. Comparison of birth weights recorded in the three UK studies are revealing, although there are methodological and sample size differences between them. Donovan's study (1977) (experimental mean birth weight = 3.17 kg; control = 3.18 kg) and the present study (experimental = 3.19 kg; control = 3.16 kg) reported findings for all babies, not just first-born. MacArthur *et al.* reported findings for all babies (experimental = 3.16 kg; control = 3.13 kg) and first-born separately (experimental = 3.16 kg; control = 3.07 kg). The mean birth weight of babies in all three is remarkably consistent, with the exception of the lower weight of the control group of first-born babies in MacArthur's study. One would expect first births to be lighter than all births, and it is perhaps more surprising that the weight of the corresponding experimental group is the same as that of all births. The MacArthur study was a randomized controlled trial, but only 10 per cent of women in the intervention group recalled receiving the complete intervention. In the present study, 99 per cent of mothers reported recalling the intervention and gave their opinion of it (Power *et al.* 1989).

It could be argued that, in 'clinical' terms, a key test of an intervention is not whether it increases mean birth weight but whether it reduces the number of small-for-dates or low birth weight babies under some arbitrary level, for example 2.5 kg. In this study 9 per cent of experimental group babies and 8 per cent of the controls were below 2.5 kg, and this can be compared with similar findings of 10 and 9 per cent reported in experimental and control groups in Donovan's (1977) study.

# Conclusions

There is sufficient evidence to support the view that personalized anti-smoking interventions in pregnancy have a positive impact on cessation and reduction of tobacco consumption. Intervention inevitably has financial implications and the findings of this study suggest that attempts to stop women smoking during pregnancy, which reinforce and utilize the existing skills of midwives, may cost of the order of £300 per woman (at summer 1990). The 'crude' cost of long-term cessation is, however, approximately three-fold without any further intervention. In the shorter term up to delivery, it appears that 'clinical outcomes' in terms of gains in babies' birth weight, may be somewhat limited. Few of the actual economic costs of smoking cessation in women during pregnancy are therefore likely to be offset by savings in treating low birth weight infants at a district health authority as opposed to national level. If, however, the main aim of intervention is to help women stop smoking for their own sake and in the much longer term, reinforcement of intervention after delivery should be considered and the additional financial costs of intervention be calculated relative to years of women's lives saved due to a reduction in smoking-related diseases.

# Acknowledgements

Warm thanks to all staff of the antenatal clinics at University and City Hospitals, Nottingham and to the women who took part. Special thanks to Professor Clair Chilvers for her helpful comments on the text, and to Professors E Malcolm Symonds and R J Madeley (University of Nottingham) for their support and collaboration in the Nottingham Mothers Stop Smoking Project. Thanks also to Ruth Gell for the typescript. This study was funded by Nottingham Health Authority.

# References

Doll, R., Gray, R., Hafner, B., and Peto, R. (1980). Mortality in relation to smoking: 22 years' observations on female British doctors. *British Medical Journal*, **5th April**, 967–70.

Donovan, J. W. (1977). Randomised controlled trial of anti-smoking advice in pregnancy. *British Journal of Preventive and Social Medicine*, **31**, 6–12.

Floyd, R. L., Gunter, E., Zahniser, S. C., Kendrick, J., and Stevens, J. (1990). *Integrating prenatal smoking cessation into Public Health Programmes.* Abstracts of the 7th World Conference on Tobacco and Health, 1–5 April. Perth, Western Australia, no. 233.

Gillies, P. A., Madeley, R., and Power, L. (1987). *Smoking cessation and pregnancy— A controlled trial of the impact of new technology and friendly encouragement.* Paper presented at the 6th World Conference on Smoking and Health, 9–12

November, Tokyo/Report to Nottingham Health Authority, Department of Community Medicine and Epidemiology, University of Nottingham.

Jamrozik, K., Vessey, M., Fowler, G., Wald, N., Parker, G., and Van Vunakis, H. (1984). Controlled trial of three different anti-smoking interventions in general practice. *British Medical Journal*, **288**, 1499–503.

Lowe, J. B., Windsor, R. A., and Woodby, L. (1990). *Helping pregnant women who quit smoking during pregnancy to stay quit: a need for relapse prevention*. Paper presented at 7th World Conference on Tobacco and Health, 1–5th April. Perth, Western Australia.

MacArthur, C., Newton, J. R., and Knox, E. G. (1987). Effect of anti-smoking health education on infant size at birth: a randomised controlled trial. *British Journal of Obstetrics and Gynaecology*, **94**, 295–300.

Madeley, R. J., Gillies, P. A., Power, F. L., and Symonds, E. M. (1989). Nottingham Mothers Stop Smoking Project—Baseline Survey of Smoking in Pregnancy. *Community Medicine*, **11**, 124–30.

Power, F. L., Gillies, P. A., Madeley, R. J., and Abbott, M. (1989). Research in an antenatal clinic. *Midwifery*, **5**, 106–12.

Royal College of Physicians (1977). *Smoking or health: a report of the Royal College of Physicians*. Pitman Medical, London.

Russell, M. A. H., Wilson, C., Taylor, C., and Baker, C. D. (1979). Effect of general practitioners' advice against smoking. *British Medical Journal*, **2**, 231–5.

Ryan, P., Booth, R., Coates, D., Chapman, A., and Healy, P. (1980). *Experiences of pregnancy: report of a survey of postpartum women in Newcastle and Wollongong*. Division of Drug and Alcohol Services, Health Commission of New South Wales, Australia.

Sexton, M. and Hebel, J. R. (1984). A clinical trial of change in maternal smoking and its effect on birthweight. *Journal of the American Medical Association*, **251**, 911–15.

Shakespeare, R. and Batten, L. (1990). *Smoking in pregnancy—a district trial of the effects of a training programme for midwives*. Abstracts of the 7th World Conference on Tobacco and Health, 1–5th April. Perth, Western Australia.

Simmons, R. A. (1988). *A smoking cessation intervention for low income women*. Abstracts of the XIII World Conference on Health Education, August. Houston, Texas.

Tones, K. (1986). The methodology of health education. *Journal of the Royal Society of Medicine*, (**Suppl. 13**) **79**, 5–7.

Trent Regional Health Authority (1984). *Community Health Service Statistics 1983*. Trent Regional Health Authority, Sheffield.

Windsor, R. A. and Orleans, C. T. (1986). Guidelines and methodological standards for smoking cessation intervention research among pregnant women: improving science and art. *Health Education Quarterly*, **13**, 131–61.

Windsor, R. A., Cutter, G., Morris, J., Reese, Y., Manzella, B., Bartlett, E. E., *et al.* (1985). The effectiveness of smoking cessation methods for smokers in public health maternity clinics: a randomised trial. *American Journal of Public Health*, **75**, 1389–92.

Windsor-Richards, K. and Gillies, P. A. (1988). Racial grouping and women's experience of giving birth in hospital. *Midwifery*, **4**, 171–6.

# 16. Measuring serum cotinine to aid in smoking cessation during pregnancy and to enhance assessment of smoking-related fetal morbidity

*James E Haddow, George J Knight, and Glenn E Palomaki*

Several pregnancy outcome parameters have been extensively examined in relation to womens' smoking habits during pregnancy, including most prominently, birth weight, length of gestation, fetal viability, and late pregnancy complications. Birth weights of infants born to mothers who smoke are, on average, approximately 200 g lower than when mothers do not smoke, the infants are born slightly earlier, and there is a 30 per cent higher risk of fetal or infant death. Abruptio placentae also occurs more frequently.

Most of the studies examining these relationships have relied upon the pregnant woman's report of her smoking status, including whether or not she smokes and, if so, how many cigarettes per day. Even though this measure of exposure has yielded reproducible data from many sources, there has been speculation that a proportion of the women might have been misclassified, either because they did not tell the truth or because variations in smoking technique or type of cigarette smoked might have affected the quantity of smoke products actually inhaled and absorbed into the bloodstream. If this were the case, and if a more objective measure of cigarette smoke exposure could be found, then it might become possible to describe the impact of maternal smoking on the pregnancy outcome parameters more accurately.

Self-reporting can be unreliable, particularly if the subject is under pressure to quit for health reasons. Most importantly, however, consumption of tobacco products, even when correctly reported, can be a poor measure of inhaled dose, as smokers vary intake by the manner of smoking (e.g. length and depth of inhalation, number and size of puffs, cigarette type). Only 20–30 per cent of the variability in biochemical indices of smoking exposure is accounted for by the number of cigarettes smoked (Feyerabend *et al.* 1982; Vesey *et al.* 1982). This problem has led to the use of biochemical markers for measuring tobacco smoke intake in body fluids and gases, including thiocyanate, carboxyhaemoglobin, carbon monoxide (CO), nicotine, and cotinine. Thiocyanate, a metabolite of the hydrogen cyanide found in tobacco smoke, was employed extensively in the earlier studies and was found generally helpful in judging smoking status (Cohen and Bartsch 1979; Vogt *et al.* 1977; Dalferes *et al.* 1980; Vesey *et al.* 1982; Haley *et al.* 1983; Hill *et al.* 1983). A major drawback, however, was its relative non-specificity—thiocyanate levels can also be elevated after ingesting certain foods (Maleszewski and Boes 1955; Haley *et al.* 1983). This non-specificity makes the assay insensitive for interpreting light smoking and also produces false-positive test results (Haley *et al.* 1983). Carboxyhaemoglobin, a second biochemical measure that is directed at the CO component of tobacco smoke, has also proved helpful in epidemiological studies, but CO in the body originates from endogenous processes as well as environmental sources (Wald *et al.* 1981). Carbon monoxide has also been measured directly in expired air using portable monitors, and this approach has been found useful both for studying smoking behaviour and for demonstration purposes with patients (Vogt *et al.* 1979). The half-life of CO is only 2–4 h, however, and does not provide a reliable picture of smoking status if the individual has avoided smoking during the preceding day (National Research Council 1981). Nicotine has been measured extensively in research studies, usually under carefully controlled conditions, and such measurements have been effective in providing insights into both smoking behaviour and nicotine metabolism (Wilcox *et al.* 1979; Feyerabend *et al.* 1982; Benowitz *et al.* 1983*a*; Greenberg *et al.* 1984; Wald *et al.* 1984*a*). Nicotine's half-life in serum, however, is only about 30 min, making it relatively ineffective for assessing chronic smoking behaviour because of its rapid disappearance when smoking is stopped (Benowitz *et al.* 1983*b*). Nictoine is rapidly metabolized in the liver to cotinine, a chemically stable, metabolically inactive compound with a circulating half-life of about 1 day (Benowitz *et al.* 1983*b*). Figure 16.1 displays the chemical structures of nicotine and cotinine; the two chemical structures differ only by a double-bonded oxygen.

Cotinine levels are relatively constant in a given individual, making cotinine suitable for assessing smoking behaviour during the previous few days. Cotinine is very stable in serum, saliva, and urine samples, and resists degradation at room temperature for prolonged periods of time; for this reason biological samples can be shipped unrefrigerated and stored in a freezer for future reference. No plant or other product that people ingest or inhale is known to contain nicotine or cotinine, thereby reducing the chances of false-positive or

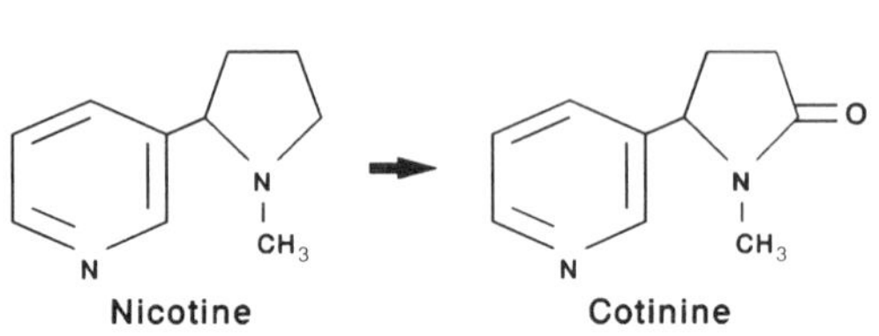

**Fig. 16.1.** The chemical structures of nicotine and cotinine.

confounding results. Collectively, these factors make cotinine the best of the available smoking markers for general population use (Zeidenberg *et al.* 1977; Wilcox *et al.* 1979; Wald *et al.* 1981; Benowitz *et al.* 1983*b*; Haley *et al.* 1983; Hill *et al.* 1983; Greenberg *et al.* 1984; Sepkovic and Haley 1985) and, on this basis, cotinine was selected as the biochemical measure of tobacco smoke intake for all of the pregnancy studies described in this chapter.

Cotinine has been measured by high performance liquid chromatography (Watson 1977; Saunders and Blume 1981), gas chromatography (Jacob *et al.* 1981; Thompson *et al.* 1982), radioimmunoassay (Knight *et al.* 1985; Langone and Van Vunakis 1982), and enzyme-linked immunosorbent assay (ELISA; Bjercke *et al.* 1986, 1987). The chromatographic procedures are highly specific and sensitive, but involve elaborate preparation steps, which are expensive and time-consuming. The immunoassays do not require preliminary steps prior to analysis, are relatively inexpensive, and can be carried out on a large number of samples. Furthermore, the immunoassays that have been developed for cotinine are highly specific (i.e. they manifest negligible cross-reactivity with nicotine or other substances) and are capable of measuring, without difficulty, the inhaled products of even one cigarette daily (Langone and Van Vunakis 1982; Benowitz *et al.* 1983*b*; Knight *et al.* 1985; Bjercke *et al.* 1986, 1987). Cotinine is also now being used as a measure of exposure to environmental tobacco smoke in non-smokers (Wald *et al.* 1984*b*).

Immunoassays have been described using both monoclonal and polyclonal antisera (Langone and Van Vunakis 1982; Knight *et al.* 1985; Bjercke *et al.* 1986, 1987). While monoclonal antibody might appear to be a preferable source for immunoassay development, it is restricted in availability, and the cost of developing another such antibody would be prohibitive. The alternative of using polyclonal antisera for ELISA development has not been a reasonable option until recently because of 'bridge' recognition in conventional antisera. This phenomenon occurs because the chemical bridge that links the cotinine to a carrier protein to form an immunogen is identical to that which links the cotinine to an enzyme or solid phase. The cotinine/conjugate reacts with the anti-bridge antibodies elicited by the immunogen and manifests greater affinity for the antiserum than cotinine itself and causes a loss of sensitivity, high background noise, and a shallow dose–response curve (Corrie and Hunter 1981).

When the programme to study tobacco smoke intake in pregnancy began, immunoassay reagents for measuring cotinine were not available either commercially or from other sources. Therefore rabbit antiserum was produced, using as the immunogen a conjugate of cotinine (the hapten) coupled via a chemical bridge to keyhole limpet haemocyanin (the carrier protein). Cotinine is a small molecule that, by itself, is not recognized as foreign by an animal. When an animal is injected with the conjugate, however, its immune system produces a family of antibodies with specific affinity for different portions of the conjugate molecule, including some that recognize the areas where cotinine is attached. The antiserum subsequently produced by the rabbit contained antibodies not only against cotinine itself, but also against the chemical bridge and, once these were removed, it became possible to design a radioimmuno-assay with satisfactory performance characteristics. Because cotinine is so similar structurally to nicotine, the antiserum was also absorbed to remove those cross-reacting antibodies. Figure 16.2 displays a standard curve of cotinine measurements in the range of 10–800 ng/ml (25–80 per cent bind-ing), after the antiserum was absorbed and the assay optimized.

Initially, the reliability of pregnant women's answers to a question about their cigarette smoking habits was examined. The source of the study popu-lation was a statewide prenatal screening programme for neural tube defects in which serum samples were sent for alpha-fetoprotein (AFP) testing from 60 per cent of the state's pregnancies. The laboratory slip for ordering the AFP test contained a question that asked if the woman smoked cigarettes and, if so, how many she smoked per day. The answer to the smoking question is now completed by 95 per cent of the women. Cotinine measurements were performed on a cohort of the serum samples without the womens' knowledge, after the samples had been coded for confidentiality. Answers to the yes/no question about smoking were highly reliable: only 3 per cent of the women who identified themselves as non-smokers had cotinine levels in the range of smokers (Haddow *et al.* 1986). Conversely, 3 per cent of women who declared themselves as smokers had cotinine levels consistent with not smoking. Clerical or transcription errors might explain an occasional misclassification in both of these groups, and most of the remainder from self-reported non-smokers are likely because of not telling the truth. The lower cotinine values in a remain-

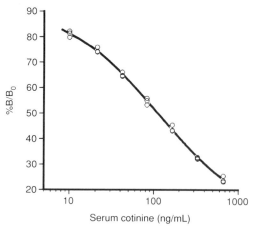

**Fig. 16.2.** Standard curve for a cotinine radioimmunoassay designed to measure absorption of nicotine in cigarette smokers. The vertical axis represents the [125]I count (B) bound by each standard, expressed as a per cent of the [125]I count (B$_0$) bound by the zero standard.

ing few of the smokers are more difficult to explain. In some, the laboratory form was filled out some weeks earlier and they might have stopped smoking in the interim. It is also possible that nicotine might be metabolized differently in a small percentage of individuals. We found a 10 ng/ml concentration of cotinine in serum to be a reasonable demarcation point between smokers and non-smokers. In Fig. 16.3, distributions of cotinine concentrations are displayed for women who report either smoking at least one cigarette per day or who report not smoking. Non-smokers who are passively exposed to tobacco smoke rarely have cotinine concentrations higher than 5 ng/ml, while smokers of even one or two cigarettes per day consistently have serum cotinine concentrations above that level. The data indicate that, for screening purposes, answers to a yes/no question about cigarette smoking are highly reliable in the pregnant population.

The smoking patterns of pregnant women who smoke cigarettes were also compared with non-pregnant adult smokers by analysing reported numbers of cigarettes smoked and serum cotinine levels. The other adults were sampled during routine group health examinations in the workplace. The differences between the two populations that appear worthy of noting are summarized in Table 16.1. The median serum cotinine level is lower for pregnant women, and this lower value appears to result both from fewer cigarettes smoked and from a smaller serum cotinine concentration per cigarette smoked. The cotinine per cigarette ratio in the pregnant women is significantly lower than ratios for the non-pregnant women and the men ($P = 0.03$ using a two-sided $t$-test on the log transformed ratios). This phenomenon might be explained by decreased inhalation or absorption, altered metabolism of nicotine, or dilution of cotinine by increased circulatory volume. Smoking habits and serum

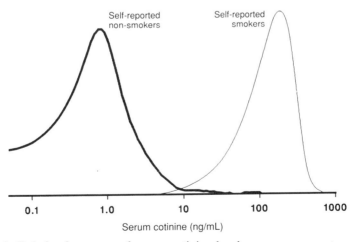

**Fig. 16.3.** Relative frequency of serum cotinine levels among pregnant women who identified themselves either as cigarette smokers or as non-smokers.

**Table 16.1** Cigarettes smoked and serum cotinine levels among pregnant and non-pregnant adult smokers

|  | Cigarettes smoked/day | | Median serum cotinine level (ng/ml) | Median serum cotinine/cigarette (ng/ml)* |
|---|---|---|---|---|
|  | *n* | mean |  |  |
| Pregnant women | 1572 | 15 | 137 | 9.4 |
| Non-pregnant women | 64 | 22 | 305 | 12.4 |
| Men | 40 | 30 | 372 | 12.8 |

* Designates the median of individually calculated ratios.

cotinine levels during pregnancy differ significantly from the non-pregnant adult population.

Next, the dose–response relationship between numbers of cigarettes smoked and serum cotinine concentrations was examined. The two measures were correlated, with a linear dose–response (Fig. 16.4). Individual cotinine measurements were, however, widely scattered at all intervals of daily cigarette consumption, with only a slight indication that some of the women might be under-reporting the numbers of cigarettes smoked. For example, a significant proportion of women reporting five cigarettes per day had serum cotinine values in the upper quartile for all smokers, but, to counterbalance

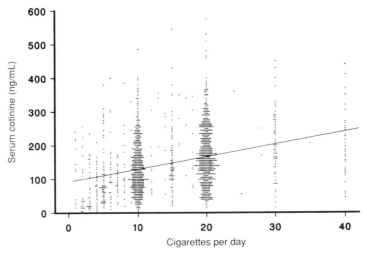

**Fig. 16.4** Scatterplot of serum cotinine concentrations in relation to self-reported numbers of cigarettes smoked.

this, a significant proportion of women smoking 20 cigarettes per day had serum cotinine values in the lowest quartile. These distributions were consistent with the hypothesis that smoking technique, type of cigarette, or some other variable might have a substantial influence on the actual absorption of cigarette smoke products.

Average birth weights in the study population were 230 g lower when the women smoked, whether defined by the yes/no answer or by serum cotinine measurements. As one way to evaluate the strength of the relation between numbers of cigarettes smoked and birth weight versus the serum cotinine level and birth weight, two intervals of cigarettes smoked (10 and 20/day) were first selected and, at each interval, birth weight examined in relation to serum cotinine level. An association between birth weight and serum cotinine concentration was found at both of the cigarette intervals (Fig. 16.5), with a 300 g birth weight differential among women smoking 10 cigarettes per day and a 200 g differential among those smoking 20 cigarettes per day. As a cross-check, two levels of serum cotinine of approximately 100 and 200 ng/ml were selected and birth weight examined in relation to cigarettes smoked. The range of birth weight differences was 25 and 75 g, respectively. Serum cotinine levels thus appeared to add information relevant to birth weight, once daily cigarette intake was known, but factoring in cigarette intake once cotinine level was known appeared to add little information.

Table 16.2 contains a more comprehensive analysis of birth weight, based

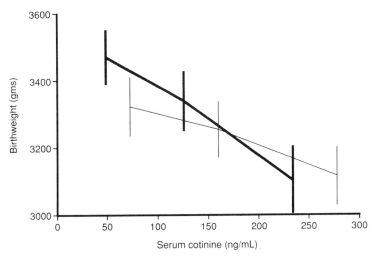

**Fig. 16.5** Serum cotinine concentrations in relation to birth weight at two intervals of self-reported cigarette smoking (10 and 20 per day). The heavy line represents the serum cotinine/birth weight relationship at 10 cigarettes per day. The lighter line represents that relationship at 20 cigarettes per day. Vertical bars indicate 95 per cent confidence intervals for birth weight stratified into three groups of equal size.

**Table 16.2** Number of women, mean birth weight and percentage of birth weights ≤ 2800 g according to reported number of cigarettes smoked each day and serum cotinine

| Serum continine Category (mean) (ng/ml) | | Number of cigarettes/day | | | | | | |
|---|---|---|---|---|---|---|---|---|
| | | 0 (0) | 1–7 (4.2) | 8–12 (9.9) | 13–17 (15.0) | 18–24 (20.0) | ≥ 25 (34.1) | All |
| 0–24 | No. women | 2759 | 62 | 32 | 4 | 15 | 2 | 2874 |
| (1) | Mean BWT | 3508 | 3475 | 3633 | 3548 | 3598 | 3231 | 3509 |
| | Per cent ≤ 2800 g | 7.5 | 6.5 | 3.1 | 0 | 0 | 0 | 7.4 |
| 25–69 | No. women | 44 | 62 | 71 | 9 | 51 | 8 | 245 |
| (48) | Mean BWT | 3329 | 3358 | 3419 | 3511 | 3286 | 3345 | 3360 |
| | Per cent ≤ 2800 g | 11.4 | 14.5 | 8.5 | 0 | 15.7 | 0 | 11.4 |
| 70–137 | No. women | 35 | 73 | 126 | 37 | 117 | 20 | 408 |
| (103) | Mean BWT | 3429 | 3367 | 3430 | 3262 | 3313 | 3507 | 3373 |
| | Per cent ≤ 2800 g | 17.1 | 8.2 | 7.1 | 10.8 | 11.1 | 10 | 9.8 |
| 138–153 | No. women | 8 | 14 | 26 | 6 | 41 | 5 | 100 |
| (145) | Mean BWT | 3625 | 3472 | 3232 | 3044 | 3260 | 3455 | 3293 |
| | Per cent ≤ 2800 g | 0 | 7.1 | 11.5 | 50.0 | 26.8 | 0 | 18 |
| 154–284 | No. women | 20 | 30 | 132 | 30.0 | 194 | 64 | 470 |
| (209) | Mean BWT | 3277 | 3225 | 3131 | 3136 | 3195 | 3154 | 3173 |
| | Per cent ≤ 2800 g | 15.0 | 20.0 | 22.0 | 30.0 | 14.9 | 20.3 | 18.9 |
| > 284 | No. women | 5 | 6 | 23 | 10 | 54 | 16 | 114 |
| (350) | Mean BWT | 3594.0 | 3230 | 3083 | 2890 | 3065 | 2943 | 3068 |
| | Per cent ≤ 2800 g | 0 | 33.3 | 17.4 | 60.0 | 27.8 | 31.3 | 28.1 |
| All | No. women | 2871 | 247 | 410 | 96 | 472 | 115 | 4211 |
| | Mean BWT | 3503 | 3376 | 3316 | 3206 | 3235 | 3214 | 3433 |
| | Per cent ≤ 2800 g | 7.7 | 11.3 | 12.7 | 22.9 | 16.0 | 17.4 | 10.0 |

From Haddow *et al*. 1987. Reprinted with permission of the *British Journal of Obstetrics and Gynaecology*.
  BWT, birth weight.

on a two-way analysis of variance over the entire range of cigarette consumption (exposure) versus serum cotinine level (absorption) (Haddow *et al*. 1987). Women who smoke ≥ 25 cigarettes per day (the 2.7 per cent of women with the greatest cigarette consumption) have infants 289 g lighter than non-smokers. Women with cotinine levels ≥ 284 ng/ml (the 2.7 per cent of women with the highest cotinine values) have infants 441 g lighter than women with the lowest cotinine levels. According to these analyses, serum cotinine levels are more closely associated with birth weight than cigarettes smoked, thereby further supporting the appropriateness of using serum cotinine measurements for studying cigarette smoking in pregnancy. At the time when data about the pregnant womens' smoking habits were being collected for this study, the yes/ no answer about smoking had not yet been placed on the AFP order form. The only question asked was: 'How many cigarettes per day do you smoke?' This study discovered that non-smokers tended not to answer the question, as proven by measuring serum cotinine levels from non-responders. It was this insight that prompted rephrasing of the question about smoking. The rate of smoking among women in the population during the second trimester, taking into account the non-responders, is actually 23 per cent.

During the process of measuring serum cotinine levels during pregnancy the opportunity arose to compare fetal serum cotinine levels with paired maternal cotinine levels in five women who smoked cigarettes and whose pregnancies required percutaneous umbilical blood sampling procedures (PUBS) (Donnenfeld *et al.* 1989). The PUBS procedures were carried out later in pregnancy (21–31 weeks gestation) than samples from the AFP screening programme, but the maternal serum cotinine levels appeared comparable. In this small study, fetal cotinine levels averaged 88 per cent of the maternal cotinine levels, suggesting the following possibilities:

(1) nicotine crossed the placenta and was metabolized to cotinine;
(2) cotinine crossed the placenta following its production in the maternal liver;
(3) both nicotine and cotinine crossed the placenta.

Changes in fetal physiological measurements immediately following maternal smoking provide indirect evidence that nicotine crosses the placenta.

There was also an opportunity to examine serum cotinine levels among a cohort of 1508 women in the AFP screening population who declared themselves to be non-smokers and to analyse those levels in relation to birth weight (Haddow *et al.* 1988). To measure the cotinine levels in this subset of second trimester pregnant women, it was necessary to design a modified cotinine radioimmunoassay, with a standard curve that spanned a range from 0.5 ng/ml to 20 ng/ml (Knight *et al.* 1989) (Fig. 16.6). In this population, 29 of the cotinine values (1.9 per cent) were $\geq 10$ ng/ml, and these were classified as being consistent with at least occasional smoking. Once these were removed, 1231 women remained who had viable singleton pregnancies and for whom it was possible to obtain complete demographic, biophysical, and birth weight information. Only 19 of these remaining pregnancies (1.5 per cent) were associated with serum cotinine levels between 5.0 and 9.9 ng/ml. Evidence for environmental tobacco smoke (ETS) absorption (serum cotinine level 1.0–9.9 ng/ml) was present in 31.4 per cent of the study population and, among those women, the crude mean birth weight was 107 g lower than the

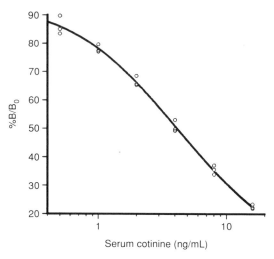

**Fig. 16.6.** Standard curve for a cotinine radioimmunoassay designed to measure absorption of nicotine in non-smokers. The vertical axis represents the $^{125}$I count (B) bound by each standard, expressed as a per cent of the $^{125}$I count ($B_0$) bound by the zero standard.

mean birth weight from the women with cotinine values < 1.0 ng/ml (95 per cent confidence interval (CI) −173 to −35 g). This difference remained after applying a multivariate analysis that included the major birth weight-associated covariates. Earlier studies relying upon non-smoking womens' estimates of exposure to environmental tobacco smoke have yielded conflicting information, with more recent studies finding an association between ETS exposure and birth weight. The extent of the birth weight difference between exposed and unexposed women in this study population was surprising, however. Even with the multivariate analysis, some other factor associated with birth weight that might have segregated with the mother's serum cotinine levels cannot be ruled out. Figure 16.7 presents the relationship between serum cotinine levels and birth weight in both passive and active smokers. This relationship is not a straight line function and may indicate that more than one mechanism is involved in influencing birth weight among the women exposed either actively or passively to cigarette smoke products.

Having found that serum cotinine measurements could be interpreted reliably to indicate tobacco smoke absorption, we designed a randomized intervention trial aimed at smoking cessation, to be carried out in the population of pregnant women enrolling for AFP screening during the second trimester, the primary goal of which was to increase birth weight. The trial superimposed a minimum intervention protocol upon routine prenatal care activities in a large population of pregnancies, receiving services from many health

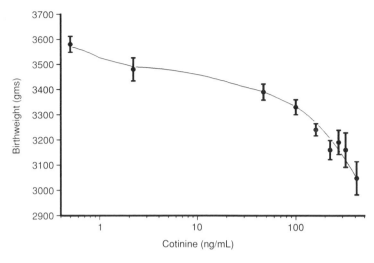

**Fig. 16.7.** The relationship between serum cotinine and birth weight, including both pregnant women who do not smoke (both passively exposed and not exposed) and pregnant women who smoke. The vertical lines with each circle are 95 per cent confidence intervals and the cotinine measurements are plotted on a logarithmic scale.

care providers. A large proportion of pregnancies throughout the United States and Western Europe now receive second trimester AFP screening through well organized, centralized programmes and it was felt that these programmes might also be suitable for orchestrating systematic smoking cessation activities. By the second trimester, when AFP screening is carried out, most women who will stop smoking on their own have already done so, and those who might stop smoking with added prompting still have the motivation that they can influence their infant's growth *in utero*.

During the trial, 139 physicians in the State of Maine allowed both randomization of their patients who, at the time of AFP screening, smoked 10 or more cigarettes per day and measurement of serum cotinine levels on those selected for interventions. Women were randomized individually, and so both cases and controls would be likely to be found in all of the physicians' practices. The serum cotinine measurements were interpreted in the context of how birth weight might be affected, and a report of this interpretation (Fig. 16.8) was sent to the physician, along with a smoking cessation guide, to be shared with the patient. A second blood sample for serum cotinine measurement was sought from the woman via the physician 1 month later, and an interpreted report of that measurement (Fig. 16.9) was also transmitted to the physician, again to share with the patient. This second report was analysed in relation to the first, as a way to help the woman judge her progress. No further intervention was attempted. The serum sample obtained from the non-

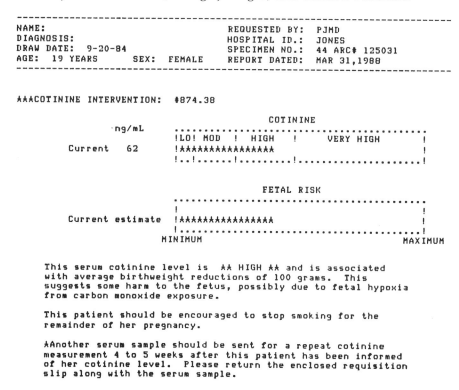

```
--------------------------------------------------------------------
NAME:                                REQUESTED BY: PJMD
DIAGNOSIS:                           HOSPITAL ID.: JONES
DRAW DATE:   9-20-84                 SPECIMEN NO.: 44 ARC# 125031
AGE:  19 YEARS       SEX:  FEMALE    REPORT DATED:  MAR 31,1988
--------------------------------------------------------------------


***COTININE INTERVENTION:   #874.38

                                              COTININE
               ·ng/mL          ..................................................
                               !LO! MOD !  HIGH   !     VERY HIGH            !
          Current   62         !**************************                   !
                               !..!.......!..........!...................!


                                            FETAL RISK
                               ..................................................
                               !                                             !
          Current estimate     !**************************                   !
                               !.............................................!
                            MINIMUM                                   MAXIMUM
```

This serum cotinine level is  ** HIGH ** and is associated
with average birthweight reductions of 100 grams. This
suggests some harm to the fetus, possibly due to fetal hypoxia
from carbon monoxide exposure.

This patient should be encouraged to stop smoking for the
remainder of her pregnancy.

*Another serum sample should be sent for a repeat cotinine
measurement 4 to 5 weeks after this patient has been informed
of her cotinine level. Please return the enclosed requisition
slip along with the serum sample.

**Fig. 16.8.** Specimen laboratory report of a pregnant woman's serum cotinine measurement, to be used by her physician as an aid in smoking cessation activities.

intervention group for AFP screening was frozen, and the cotinine level measured after delivery. No contact was made with women in the non-intervention group, and no follow-up blood samples were sought.

Overall, 2848 women smoking 10 or more cigarettes per day were enrolled in the study and 2700 singleton viable pregnancies remained for analysis of birth weight after follow-up of pregnancy outcome was complete (outcome data were available for 97 per cent of the randomized women). Applying an 'intention to treat' analysis to the patients attending the offices of the 70 physicians who most effectively completed the intervention protocol (as judged by obtaining a repeat blood sample for the follow-up cotinine estimation), intervention led to a significant 66 g increase in mean birth weight ($P = 0.03$; 95 per cent CI +9 to +123 g) and to a 30 per cent reduction in the rate of low birth weight ($P = 0.08$) when compared to controls receiving care from those same offices (Haddow *et al.* 1991). Among patients attending the offices of the remaining 69 physicians, intervention had no significant effect (Fig. 16.10).

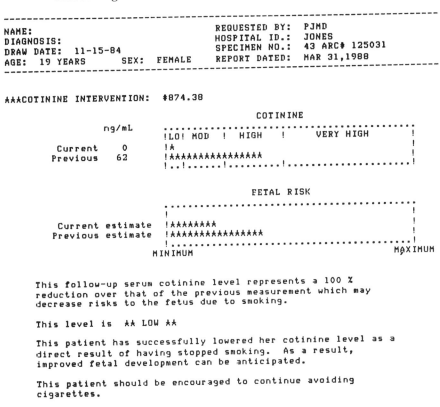

```
------------------------------------------------------------------
NAME:                         REQUESTED BY:  PJMD
DIAGNOSIS:                    HOSPITAL ID.:  JONES
DRAW DATE:  11-15-84          SPECIMEN NO.:  43 ARC# 125031
AGE:  19 YEARS    SEX: FEMALE REPORT DATED:  MAR 31,1988
------------------------------------------------------------------


***COTININE INTERVENTION:  #874.38
                                              COTININE
                                 ............................................
              ng/mL              !LO! MOD !  HIGH  !   VERY HIGH           !
     Current       0             !*                                        !
     Previous     62             !*****************                        !
                                 !..!......!.........!....................!


                                            FETAL RISK
                                 ............................................
                                 !                                        !
     Current estimate            !*******                                 !
     Previous estimate           !***************                         !
                                 !........................................!
                                 MINIMUM                          MAXIMUM
```

This follow-up serum cotinine level represents a 100 %
reduction over that of the previous measurement which may
decrease risks to the fetus due to smoking.

This level is  ** LOW **

This patient has successfully lowered her cotinine level as a
direct result of having stopped smoking.  As a result,
improved fetal development can be anticipated.

This patient should be encouraged to continue avoiding
cigarettes.

**Fig. 16.9.** Specimen follow-up laboratory report of a pregnant woman's repeat serum cotinine measurement, approximately 1 month after the first.

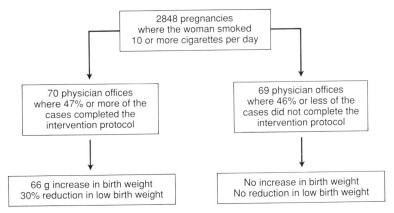

**Fig. 16.10.** Summary of results from a randomized intervention trial, in which serum cotinine measurements were employed to assist smoking cessation activities during pregnancy.

Results of this study were encouraging, in that 75 per cent of all physicians in Maine were willing to participate in this trial, and half of those participating carried out the intervention protocol effectively, even though that protocol had not been proven to influence smoking habits. Furthermore, both mean birth weight and the rate of low birth weight appeared to be favourably influenced when the intervention protocol was adhered to. The intervention protocol was not expensive, nor was it disruptive to the office routine. The data from this study indicate that this type of approach to smoking cessation in pregnancy might be successfully applied elsewhere, utilizing existing AFP screening programmes. In addition, the impression was gained that this approach to smoking cessation might be more effective, both in relation to numbers of physicians participating and to numbers of physicians adhering to the protocol, now that this strategy has been found successful. There is much to be said in favour of managing smoking cessation activities during pregnancy from a central source. Using this approach, women can be reached more systematically and instruments of proven effectiveness can be used. Furthermore, impact can be monitored. Whether the cotinine-assisted intervention protocol or some other intervention protocol proves to be more effective is ultimately less important than having a well organized delivery system.

## Acknowledgement

The randomized trial described in this text was totally supported by NIH Grant # R01 HD 18274–01.

## References

Benowitz, N. L., Hall, S. M., Herning, R. I., Jacob, P., Jones, R. T., and Osman, A. L. (1983*a*). Smokers of low-yield cigarettes do not consume less nicotine. *New England Journal of Medicine*, **309**, 139–42.

Benowitz, N. L., Kuyt, F., Jacob, P., Jones, R. T., and Osman, A. L. (1983*b*). Cotinine disposition and effects. *Clinical Pharmacology and Therapeutics*, **34**, 604–11.

Bjercke, R. J., Cook, G., Rychlik, N., Gjika, H. B., Van Vunakis, H., and Langone, J. J. (1986). Stereospecific monoclonal antibodies to nicotine and cotinine and their use in enzyme-linked immunosorbent assays. *Journal of Immunological Methods*, **90**, 203–13.

Bjercke, R. J., Cook, G., and Langone, J. J. (1987). Comparison of monoclonal and polyclonal antibodies to cotinine in nonisotopic and isotopic immunoassays. *Journal of Immunological Methods*, **96**, 239–46.

Cohen, J. D. and Bartsch, G. E. (1979). A comparison between carboxyhemoglobin and serum thiocyanate determinations as indicators of cigarette smoking. *American Journal of Public Health*, **69**, 1272–4.

Corrie, J. E. T. and Hunter, W. M. (1981). 125-Iodinated tracers for hapten specific radioimmunoassay. *Methods in Enzymology*, **738**, 79–112.

Dalferes, E. R., Webber, L. S., Radhakrishramurthy, B., and Berenson, G. S.

(1980). Continuous flow (AutoAnalyzer 1) analysis for plasma thiocyanate as an index to tobacco smoking. *Clinical Chemistry*, **26**, 493–5.

Donnenfeld, A. E., Pulkkinen, A. J., Palomaki, G. E., Knight, G. J., and Haddow, J. E. (1989). Serum cotinine levels in non-pregnant adult smokers, pregnant mothers who smoke, and exposed fetuses. *American Journal of Human Genetics*, **45(Suppl.)**, A257.

Feyerabend, C., Higgenbottam, T., and Russell, M. A. H. (1982). Nicotine concentrations in urine and saliva of smokers and non-smokers. *British Medical Journal*, **284**, 1002–4.

Greenberg, R. A., Haley, N. J., Etzel, R. A., and Loda, F. A. (1984). Measuring the exposure of infants to tobacco smoke. Nicotine and cotinine in urine and saliva. *New England Journal of Medicine*, **310**, 1075–8.

Haddow, J. E., Palomaki, G. E., and Knight, G. J. (1986). Use of serum cotinine to assess the accuracy of self-reported non-smoking. *British Medical Journal*, **293**, 1306.

Haddow, J. E., Knight, G. J., Palomaki, G., Kloza, E. M., and Wald, N. J. (1987). Cigarette consumption and serum cotinine in relation to birthweight. *British Journal of Obstetrics and Gynaecology*, **94**, 678–81.

Haddow, J. E., Knight, G. J., Palomaki, G. E., and McCarthy, J. E. (1988). Second trimester serum cotinine levels in nonsmokers in relation to birthweight. *American Journal of Obstetrics and Gynecology*, **159**, 481–4.

Haddow, J. E., Knight, G. J., Kloza, E. M., Palomaki, G. E., and Wald, N. J. (1991). A randomized trial of cotinine-assisted intervention to reduce smoking in pregnancy and reduce low birthweight delivery. *British Journal of Obstetrics and Gynaecology*, **98**, 859–65.

Haley, N. J., Axelrad, C. M., and Tilton, K. A. (1983). Validation of self-reported smoking behavior: Biochemical analyses of cotinine and thiocyanate. *American Journal of Public Health*, **73**, 1204–7.

Hill, P., Haley, N. J., and Wynder, E. L. (1983). Cigarette smoking: Carboxyhemoglobin, plasma nicotine, cotinine, and thiocyanate vs. self-reported smoking data and cardiovascular disease. *Journal of Chronic Diseases*, **36**, 439–49.

Jacob, P., Wilson, M., and Benowitz, N. L. (1981). Improved gas chromatographic method for the determination of nicotine and cotinine in biologic fluids. *Journal of Chromatography*, **229**, 61–70.

Knight, G. J., Wylie, P., Holman, M. S., and Haddow, J. E. (1985). Improved I-125 radioimmunoassay for cotinine by selective removal of bridge antibodies. *Clinical Chemistry*, **31**, 118–21.

Knight, G. J., Palomaki, G. E., Lea, D. H., and Haddow, J. E. (1989). Exposure to environmental tobacco smoke measured by cotinine [125]I-radioimmunoassay. *Clinical Chemistry*, **35**, 1036–9.

Langone, J. J. and Van Vunakis, H. V. (1982). Radioimmunoassay of nicotine, cotinine, and alpha-(3-pyridyl)-alpha-oxo-N-methylbutylamide. *Methods in Enzymology*, **84D**, 628–40.

Maleszewski, T. F. and Boes, D. E. (1955). True and apparent thiocyanate in body fluids of smokers and non-smokers. *Journal of Applied Physiology*, **8**, 289–96.

National Research Council Committee (1981). *Medical and biologic effects of environmental pollutant. Carbon monoxide.* National Academy Press, Washington DC.

Saunders, J. A. and Blume, D. E. (1981). Quantitation of major tobacco alkaloids by high-performance liquid chromatography. *Journal of Chromatography*, **205**, 147–54.

Sepkovic, D. W. and Haley, N. J. (1985). Biomedical applications of cotinine quantitation in smoking related research. *American Journal of Public Health,* **75,** 663–5.

Thompson, J. A., Ho, M., and Petersen, D. R. (1982). Analyses of nicotine and cotinine in tissues by capillary gas chromatography and gas chromatography – mass spectrometry. *Journal of Chromatography,* **231,** 53–63.

Vesey, C. J., Saloojee, Y., Cole, P. V., and Russell, M. A. H. (1982). Blood carboxyhemoglobin, plasma thiocyanate, and cigarette consumption: Implications for epidemiological studies in smokers. *British Medical Journal,* **284,** 1516–18.

Vogt, T. M., Selven, S., Widdowson, G., and Hulley, S. B. (1977). Expired air carbon monoxide and serum thiocyanate as objective measures of cigarette exposure. *American Journal of Public Health,* **67,** 545–9.

Vogt, T. M., Selvin, S., and Billings, J. H. (1979). Smoking cessation program: Baseline carbon monoxide and serum thiocyanate levels as predictors of outcome. *American Journal of Public Health,* **69,** 1156–9.

Wald, N. J., Idle, M., Boreham, J., and Bailey, A. (1981). Serum cotinine levels in pipe smokers: Evidence against nicotine as cause of coronary heart disease. *Lancet,* **ii,** 775–7.

Wald, N. J., Idle, M., Boreham, J., Bailey, A., and Van Vunakis, H. (1984*a*). Urinary nicotine in cigarette and pipe smokers. *Thorax,* **39,** 365–8.

Wald, N. J., Boreham, J., Bailey, A., Ritchie, C., Haddow, J. E., and Knight, G. J. (1984*b*). Urinary cotinine as a marker of breathing other people's smoke. *Lancet,* **i,** 230–1.

Watson, I. D. (1977). Rapid analysis of nicotine and cotinine in the urine of smokers of using isocratic high-performance liquid chromatography. *Journal of Chromatography,* **143,** 203–6.

Wilcox, R. G., Hughes, J., and Roland, J. (1979). Verification of smoking history in patients after infarction using urinary nicotine and cotinine measurements. *British Medical Journal,* **ii,** 1026–8.

Zeidenberg, P., Jaffe, J. H., Kanzler, M., Levitt, M. D., Langone, J. J., and Van Vunakis, H. (1977). Nicotine: Cotinine levels in blood during cessation of smoking. *Comprehensive Psychiatry,* **18,** 92–101.

# 17. Summary and conclusions

*Robert Waller*

---

The most striking aspect of this symposium was the demonstration of the large variety of adverse effects on reproductive outcome of exposure to tobacco smoke and the different role played by its various constituents.

The topic of fecundity in relation to smoking, introduced by Dr Baird, was generally considered to have received too little attention to date and not enough was known about possible effects through the male. While smoking was far short of a method of birth control, the indications were that smoking (by the female) could account for about 10 per cent of infertility problems and, as such, it had an appreciable public health impact. The incidence of ectopic pregnancy in smoking mothers-to-be has also to be taken into account when assessing infertility and the public health implications.

The study reported by Professor Anderson on the well-known reductions in birth weight raised interesting points about interrelationships between smoking, alcohol, and other factors in birth weight reductions. Changes in the morphology of the placenta, in the placental circulation and oxygen transfer, and animal experiments on embryo growth all pointed to the noxious influence of smoking on growth of the fetus. Even the lower pre-eclampsia rate in smokers as compared with non-smokers should not be claimed as a benefit as, when pre-eclampsia did occur among smokers it was more severe and had a greater effect on perinatal mortality.

Breast-feeding and subsequent health and educational development of the child was of topical interest in relation to efforts to promote breast-feeding as well as to discourage smoking. Interest centred on the ways in which breast-feeding interacted with the many negative effects of smoking. Such interactions were evident. Features such as breast-feeding reducing or abolishing adverse effects of maternal smoking on respiratory illnesses in the children had been clarified. One possibility considered was that it could be a dose effect related to breast-feeders being lighter smokers. The relative roles of maternal smoking during pregnancy and subsequent smoking by the mother or others in the household must be considered. Opinions differed as to whether available data supported a role of environmental tobacco smoke (ETS), including that from paternal smoking, in lower respiratory tract infection among young children, or whether prenatal smoking could be the main factor. The fact that mothers who smoked during pregnancy tended to continue afterwards made it difficult to separate such features.

The analysis from the Sheffield-based multicentre study that was presented, together with a review of other epidemiological studies, pointed to a substantial role of smoking, attributable mainly to ETS (with respiratory infection playing a contributory part), in the acknowledged important relationship with Sudden Infant Death Syndrome (SIDS).

There was agreement on important public health messages for prevention, strengthening advice not to smoke during pregnancy, and strongly recommending people not to smoke in a room with an infant. One reservation about that, however, was not to deter people too much from staying in the same room with the child. This latter theme was taken further in Professor Rush's presentation on the effects on childhood health and development. The effects of smoking on height could be accounted for mainly by adjusting for social class and birth weight, and there appeared to be no paternal smoking effects over and above those linked with maternal smoking. Discussion on such points invoked the 'chicken and egg' situation, questioning whether factors such as social class were causal or were, in fact, partly markers for smoking.

Experience with recent cessation programmes in the United States and the United Kingdom led to the conclusion that there was a need to educate obstetricians further on smoking cessation advice as an integral part of pre-natal counselling. These steps had been introduced in several centres. Face-to-face advice from physicians coupled with health education yielded the best results. The modest cost was stressed, offering net benefits when set against savings in intensive health care for low birth weight babies. Further benefits to the overall health of the mother could occur from giving up smoking. A valuable step towards improving quantitative links between smoking and birth weight was demonstrated by Professor Haddow, reporting a study in which serum cotinine measurements had been linked with birth weights. The reporting back to physicians of cotinine values so that they could be shown to the patient with an explanation of their relevance, reinforced efforts for cessation. It was possible also to show the presence of cotinine in the baby's urine, collecting via absorbent material in the nappy. The demonstration of the presence of smoke components in pregnant women in front of them in a clinic was generally considered to be a valuable adjunct to cessation efforts.

A key point in the general discussion at the end of the meeting was to what extent smoking cessation efforts should be focused on the period of pregnancy. On the one hand it was seen as a window of opportunity when concern could be aroused in relation to the well-being of the baby, plus the longer-term benefits to the health of the mother and the family generally. Cessation rates achieved in the context of pregnancy were reported to be impressive in comparison with those in general settings. On the other hand there were some reservations, as there were many other things to worry about at that time and, within antenatal clinics, patients were already seen by many different people.

The important point was considered to be for the obstetrician to establish rapport with each individual, offering reassurance on all aspects and encompassing advice on smoking. Another aspect was that in some respects, for example in relation to the morphological changes demonstrated in the placenta, there was a need to avoid smoking even before conception. Thus there was support for increased efforts against smoking among children and young women. Even so it had been seen that some reduction in adverse effects on the fetus could still be obtained if smoking was not given up until part way through pregnancy, hence there would ideally be periods of action before, during and after pregnancy.

A need was recognized to look further into the more serious outcome problems. Most studies used birth weight deficits as surrogates for perinatal mortality, but clearly the size of study required for a direct examination of this was prohibitive. Links with deaths beyond the first week should be examined. Another area for investigation could be spontaneous abortions, and there was some disappointment that little had emerged to date in respect of fetal malformations.

While the main focus of the meeting had been on smoking in pregnancy and immediate effects on the fetus, wider ranging effects that could be linked either with that initial smoking or with subsequent exposure to environmental tobacco smoke had also been covered. Among these, links with SIDS attracted considerable attention.

The long-standing evidence linking parental smoking with respiratory illnesses among young children had been further supported, notably with material from the longitudinal 1970 Birth Cohort Study, and information was beginning to emerge on possible behavioural and educational deficits. In this respect too, interrelationships with socio-economic factors remained difficult to disentangle, but it was an important aspect that deserved further attention.

Many speakers had emphasized that particular attention was needed for low-income groups, among whom smoking tended to be more prevalent and who experienced greater perinatal mortality risks and poorer subsequent respiratory health among their children.

As in the two preceding symposia in the present series (Wald and Froggatt 1989; Wald and Baron 1990), bringing together a group of active research workers across a wide range of disciplines has proved very helpful in widening knowledge of the many different effects of smoking on health, in identifying needs for further research and in guiding public health strategies. There is particular concern about involuntary exposures to harmful constituents of tobacco smoke and avoidance of exposure of the fetus and young child, whether through the mother's smoking or through environmental tobacco smoke, is clearly an important public health goal, and one that could act as a spur to the wider action against smoking through all stages of life.

# References

Wald, N. and Froggatt, P. (ed.) (1989). *Nicotine, smoking, and the low tar programme.* Oxford University Press, Oxford.

Wald, N. and Baron, J. (ed.) (1990). *Smoking and hormone-related disorders.* Oxford University Press, Oxford.

# Index